How to Help
the
Children in Disasters

Fourth Edition
Karen Olness MD
Anna Mandalakas MD MS
Kristine Torjesen MD MPH
Health Frontiers

Fourth Edition published 2015 by Health Frontiers
44500 66th Avenue Way, Kenyon, Minnesota 55946 USA
Phone: 507–789–6725, Fax: 507–789–6575
E–mail: karen.olness@case.edu
www.healthfrontiers.org

Rev: Y

Publication History

Original edition published by Health Frontiers, 1998, as
"How to Help the Children in Complex Humanitarian Emergencies,"
reprinted with J&J Pediatric Institute, 1999, as "Helping the Children,
a Practical Handbook for Complex Humanitarian Emergencies."
Spanish, Albanian editions, 1999, Arabic, Chinese, 2003
Second edition published by Health Frontiers, 2006.
Third edition published by Health Frontiers, 2014.

ISBN 978–0–615–93257–6

AUTHORS

Karen Olness, MD is Professor of Pediatrics, Global Health & Diseases at Case Western Reserve University. She has had 45 years of experience in helping children in humanitarian disasters around the world. She developed a course on "Management of Humanitarian Emergencies: focus on Children and Families" in 1995, which is given annually at CASE and has been replicated more than 20 times in other areas of the world.

Anna Maria Mandalakas, MD, MS is Associate Professor of Pediatrics and Director of the Global Childhood Tuberculosis Program at Baylor College of Medicine, Houston, Texas. Her research and clinical activities involve the care of vulnerable children, including refugees, immigrants and adoptees, with a focus on infectious disease epidemiology and childhood TB-HIV. Building upon her past experiences on several continents, her current work focuses on improving outcomes for TB-HIV affected children and families in Sub-Saharan Africa.

Kristine Torjesen, MD, MPH is Associate Director, Science Facilitation, FHI 360 in Durham, North Carolina. Her current work focuses on HIV prevention research and implementation science. She spent three years in Malawi, doing HIV/AIDS research and pediatric clinical care. She spent a year in Laos as field representative of Health Frontiers and then five years as the US-based program director of the Lao residency training programs. She has lived in several other cultures around the world, including six months as a relief worker in a refugee camp in Thailand.

FOURTH EDITION ACKNOWLEDGEMENTS

Our thanks to Dr. Kathleen Clegg for a new chapter on Self Care for Relief Workers.

PREVIOUS EDITION ACKNOWLEDGEMENTS

Thanks to Bryan Watt for his photography, preparation of the book cover, layout and uploading of the book.

We thank three residents from Rainbow Babies and Children's Hospital (Dr. Jordana Hikri, Dr. Rose Lee, and Dr. Denise Lopez Domowicz) for their contributions to the chapters on Nutrition, Obstetrics, Biochemical Terrorism, Immunization, and Medical Issues.

We thank Dr. Marisa Herran for a new chapter: Triage.

Thanks to Dr. Elie Abu Jawdeh for a new chapter on Newborn Infections and Hyperbilirubinemia.

Thanks to Dr. Saleh Al Salehi for translation of the manual into Arabic, Dr. Hossain Esmaili for translation of the manual into Farsi, and Dr. Marisa Herran for translation of the manual into Spanish.

Numerous faculty and participants in the training courses on Children in Disasters have made suggestions for revising and expanding this manual. We especially thank Dr. June Brady for her thoughtful suggestions, Dr. Mary Hellerstein for her editing, Dr. Marisa Herran for literature searches and the Spanish translation, and Dr. Eva Holsinger for her chapter on sexual and gender based violence.

This manual reflects the work and advice of many. We would like to thank Dr. Frank Klamet for his expert guidance on the birthing chapter, Dr. Edith Grotberg for her expertise on resilience in children, Dr. Arnold Anderson for reviewing the first draft and Ms. Carey Schwartz for her assistance with editing. We are grateful to the American Academy of Pediatrics and the International Pediatric Association for their encouragement in the completion of this manual.

Table of Contents

1. Introduction

This manual is written for people who work in disasters and are experts in their own area, but may not be child health specialists. This is an updated version of the manual, which was originally published in 1998.

The number of disasters affecting children increased dramatically in the last decade of the twentieth century. Large disasters in 2004 and 2005, such as the man-made disasters in Sudan and the Republic of the Congo and the natural disasters of the Asian tsunami and hurricane Katrina, received media attention and an acute outpouring of aid. The recent man-made disaster in Syria has displaced two million children either to refugee camps in other countries or within Syria. The needs and the problems of children in those disasters may continue for years or a lifetime. Half of the individuals living in many disaster settings are under 15 years of age. Morbidity and mortality in disasters are highest for children under 5 years of age. It is essential that relief workers be prepared to address child health issues in disasters.

I have worked as a pediatrician-volunteer on behalf of various agencies in humanitarian emergencies for more than 40 years. My observation is that children suffer much in these situations. They suffer both acutely and over their lifetimes, because early disaster experiences often lead to long-term physical and mental health problems. Most relief workers recognize that children have special needs, but rarely do they have the experience or knowledge necessary to meet those needs. Therefore, we developed this manual for field use, in a format that we hope is short, practical and readable.

It is not always clear why programs for children in humanitarian emergencies tend to get low priority. Some possible explanations are that children have no power; they are poor advocates for themselves; and their voices are rarely heard in policy discussions. For these reasons, the needs of children are often ignored in many types of public programs throughout the world. In disasters, well-meaning workers often lack specific child health or child development expertise. They may be unaware that children are not little adults. They may not realize that children move through many different developmental stages and therefore have rapidly changing needs. They may simply be overwhelmed by the demands of the more vocal adult population.

People throughout the world emphasize that "children are the future." At the same time, adult policy makers often do not know that the brains of young children develop most rapidly in the first year of life and that most brain development is completed by age three. It is these very young children who are the most helpless, the most vulnerable, the least able to communicate what they need, and yet are at the greatest risk of suffering irreversible brain injury in disaster situations. Programs for children should have top priority in disaster settings.

Everyone who works in a disaster setting, whether they have a child health background or not, recognizes the importance of water, food, shelter and sanitation. Everyone should know how to provide for these and the other needs of children in a developmentally appropriate and nurturing manner. We hope this manual will provide some basic and useful information on how to help the children in disasters.

Karen Olness, MD
March 2014

2. Personal Preparation

Working in a disaster is usually an intense experience, which can be both rewarding and traumatic. You can never be certain about what you will encounter. Ask yourself the following questions prior to departure in order to clarify expectations and minimize the unknown.

- Why are you doing this? Possible reasons include altruism, professional interests, family history, travel interests, or escapism. Beware of the potential for travel interests to interfere with the commitment needed to work effectively in a disaster. It is possible that you could be more effective by staying at your usual workplace and helping colleagues in the disaster area. You might assist them with electronic information, sending supplies, money, and "care packages."

- Who are the players? How many agencies are involved? Who is in charge?

- What is the history of events that led to the disaster?

- What are the relevant political, ethnic, economic and cultural issues?

- Is the situation acute and recent or has the refugee or internally displaced camp existed for some time?

- What will your duties be?

- What are the personal security and health risks for you?

- Who will be your day-to-day working colleagues?

- What are the logistics? How will you get there?

- What will your accommodations be? What is the availability of food and water? Will there be opportunities to bathe?

- How will you communicate with your family, friends and colleagues at home?

- What are the anticipated problems for children? What are the usual medical problems in the region?

- Are there disease outbreaks or epidemics in process?

- What is the nutritional state of the children?

- What is the likelihood that the children have been immunized?

- Are there unaccompanied minors (children who have been separated from their families)?

We recommend obtaining as much information as possible regarding the above questions. At the same time, be prepared to tolerate uncertainty, as information may not be available in the midst of a disaster.

For packing lists, it is best to consult with those who have traveled before you to the same area, as specific items will vary by location and conditions. There are resources on the web and in print that provide comprehensive packing lists and preparation materials for international medical volunteers (see the last chapter of this manual). Listed below are additional ways to personally prepare for work in a disaster that are based on the experience of others who have succeeded.

- Do as much as possible to prevent illness in yourself and your co-workers. Get reasonable immunizations. Prepare an emergency medical bag.

- Discuss your plans with family and friends. Arrange for regular communication with them.

- Pack with attention to the children you will be seeing as well as to your own needs. Small toys, soft balls, chewing gum, crayons and paper are a few favorite items.

- Bring a sturdy laptop or electronic reader that contains helpful manuals, books and references. A brief resource list is included at the end of this manual. In case electricity for recharging your electronic is uncertain, you may bring some hard copy resources, including this manual.

- Consider bringing camping equipment, depending on the living situation anticipated for relief workers.

- Keep a focus on prevention and what can be done to eliminate the acute problems you will encounter.

- Consider what can be done in the present to minimize long-term mental health consequences among children affected by the humanitarian emergency.

- Keep a journal. Include daily notes related to what you learn and experience, as well as ideas to help prepare your successors.

3.   Self Care for Relief Workers

No one who sees a disaster is untouched by it. [1]

Disaster workers are drawn to the work for a number of reasons, but disaster work is stressful for all involved. A comprehensive stress prevention and management plan should be incorporated into the planning of a disaster response, and should not be an afterthought when problems have surfaced in the disaster response team.

Stress is normal, necessary and often productive. It is what gives us the motivation to work to make a change when things are not going well. But stress can also be destructive. The effects of stress can be cumulative, so the chronicity of the stress plays a big part in the overall effects. Many sources of stress are identifiable and some are preventable, and this chapter will highlight some of these sources of stress. In addition to maintaining the mental health and well-being of the responder, disaster responders cannot take care of others if they cannot take care of themselves. [2]

Many reactions to a disaster can be characterized as 'normal reactions to an abnormal event.' These can include physical, emotional, cognitive and behavioral symptoms. Physical symptoms of stress include increased heart rate, blood pressure and respiratory rate. Gastrointestinal distress such as nausea, vomiting and diarrhea can occur, resulting in weight loss, or weight gain can occur. Other physical symptoms include tremor, sweating, headaches, back pain and a decreased resistance to infection.

Emotional symptoms of stress include feeling vulnerable, especially if the work involves a potential threat to the disaster worker. At the other extreme, disaster responders can feel heroic, or invulnerable, which could cloud their judgment and decision making in a disaster. Anxiety, fear, anger, and sadness are all normal responses to the stressful situations that can be encountered in a disaster including "tremendous loss of life, serious injuries, missing and separated families and destruction of whole areas." [3] Empathy is built on the foundation of the responder's ability to identify with the victims, but if taken to an extreme this identification can be immobilizing. Cognitive symptoms can include impairment in memory, disorientation or confusion, difficulty concentrating, loss of objectivity and difficulty making decisions. Behavioral stress reactions can include a change in eating or sleeping patterns, use of alcohol or other drugs, unwillingness to leave the scene until the work is done, angry outbursts, frequent arguments, social withdrawal or use of humor.

Disaster responders can develop conditions such as burnout, compassion fatigue or secondary traumatic stress reactions, sometimes referred to as secondary victimization or vicarious victimization or vicarious trauma. Burnout is a syndrome of physical and emotional exhaustion, often accompanied by a change in attitude toward the work. Burnout develops gradually, and can occur in any work setting, but is thought to be due to the unrelenting demands of one's occupation. Help can be as simple as taking time off from the work setting, or being provided with increased support in the workplace.

Unlike burnout, compassion fatigue and secondary traumatic stress often occur suddenly and without warning. Compassion fatigue can include symptoms of apathy, lowered self-esteem, and preoccupation with the trauma, as well as anxiety, guilt, numbing, anger, sadness and hypersensitivity, impatience, irritability, hypervigilance and anger at God. [4] Secondary victimization or vicarious trauma involves a cluster of symptoms that are similar to those who experienced the primary trauma, meaning those who are directly traumatized. These reactions can appear suddenly and in response to the survivors' traumatic experiences. Unlike burnout, secondary or vicarious trauma can result in changes in basic areas such as sense of trust, sense of control, self-esteem and capacity for intimacy, much as occurs in acute and post-traumatic stress reactions in victims of primary trauma. [5]

Stress prevention and management can operate at the individual as well as organizational levels. Individual approaches can involve managing the workload by setting priorities, and making sure that the plan is realistic. Maintaining as balanced a lifestyle as possible is important. This includes regular exercise, nutritious meals and adequate sleep. However, in the chaos of acute disaster, exercise, meals and sleep are rarely regular.

Contact with family and friends from home should be maintained. Individuals can identify and employ stress reduction techniques that work for them, such as practicing mindfulness, journaling or engaging in relaxation exercises, all of which could be done anywhere. On an organizational level, it is helpful if the management/leadership of the responder organization has an explicit chain of command. The purpose of the disaster response should be explicitly stated, with clearly defined roles for individuals involved in the disaster response. Responders should be oriented and trained by those already doing the work. Work responsibilities should be updated regularly. Defined work shifts with briefings at the beginning and end of shifts can support communication and enforce time off from the work. Sometimes alternating assignments from more stressful to less stressful tasks is necessary. A 'buddy system' of stress monitoring and mutual support is useful and one way to regularly assess workers' functioning. An exit plan can also be a support, allowing an opportunity for processing of the experience. Responders should be given information about common reactions to reentry back home after work in a disaster. Disaster response workers should be given opportunities to provide feedback and constructive criticism about the intervention efforts. Finally, responders can be given formal recognition for their service.

In summary, individual level and organizational level interventions aimed at preventing secondary or vicarious trauma can allow individuals to participate in disaster response, caring for themselves so they will be able to care for those affected by the disaster.

References

1.   Hartsough, DM and Myers, DG. Disaster Work and Mental Health: Prevention and Control of Stress Among Workers. Rockville, Maryland: National Institute of Mental Health, 1985.

2.   Merlino, JP: Rescuing Ourselves, in Disaster Psychiatry: Readiness, Evaluation and Treatment. Edited by Stoddard FJ, Pandya, A and Katz, C. Arlington, Virginia, American Psychiatric Publishing, 2011.

3.   Centers for Disease Control and Prevention: Emergency Preparedness and the Response: Coping with a Disaster or Traumatic Event: Atlanta, GA, Centers for Disease Control and Prevention, 2010a.

4.   Figley, CR (ed): Treating Compassion Fatigue (Routledge Psychosocial Stress Series). New York, Routledge, 2002.

5.   Quitangan, G and Evces, M (ed): Vicarious Trauma and Disaster Mental health: Understanding Risks and Promoting Resilience, New York, Routledge, 2015.

4. What, Why, Where, Who

Disasters can be defined in several ways. An objective definition is that disasters involve the destruction of property, cause injury and/or loss of life and affect large populations. A more subjective definition is that disasters exceed the capacity of a community to function normally, thus creating the need for outside assistance.

Historically, disasters are described in distinct categories such as natural or man-made. Man-made disasters include those that are technological in nature and complex humanitarian emergencies (CHEs):

- **Natural disasters:** floods, typhoons, tsunamis, earthquakes ...

- **Technological disasters:** industrial, chemical, radioactive ...

- **CHEs**: civil conflict, economic collapse, population displacement ...

A more modern perspective on disasters acknowledges the overlap that occurs between these distinct categories. We now recognize that common problems underlie the extent to which an event can or will lead to a disaster. During periods of extreme stress, critical gaps in a country's infrastructure are most easily exposed. Frequently, the public health system proves to be the weakest link. Hence, when an event does occur, the country is unable to respond effectively and a disaster results.

Socio-political and economic dynamics have become enmeshed with disasters during the post-cold war period. Less industrialized countries frequently spend a large portion of their Gross National Product (GNP) in the immediate response to a disaster, leaving few resources for recovery and rehabilitation. Ultimately, these countries become unable to respond to future disaster situations. For example, a natural drought preceded the war and civil strife that occurred in Somalia in 1980. It was late in the crisis when the international community recognized the need for extensive humanitarian assistance.

CHEs are disaster situations that involve a myriad of political, military, economic and/or natural constraints. They combine internal conflict with large-scale displacement of people and economic, social and political instability. As the total number of disasters has risen over the past 20 years, the proportion due to CHEs has dramatically increased. During the 1980s, there were 4–6 complex humanitarian emergencies each year. Since 1990 there have been between 20 and 30 complex humanitarian emergencies each year. During the same period, 30–50 major natural disasters have occurred annually. Each week there is at least one natural or man-made disaster that requires substantial external assistance.

POPULATIONS AFFECTED

The victims in disasters tend to be large populations, vulnerable groups, minority ethnic groups or cultures on the brink of extinction. Vulnerable groups are sub-populations that are particularly prone to illness and malnutrition such as infants, pregnant and lactating women, the elderly and the handicapped. Common terms used to describe different populations in disasters are refugees, internally displaced persons and unaccompanied minors.

- **Refugees:** individuals who have been forced to leave their own country.

- **Displaced persons:** individuals who have been forced to leave their homes but remain within their own country.

- **Unaccompanied minors:** children who have been separated from their parents or adult caretakers.

During the last two decades, it is estimated that disasters adversely affected 800 million people and inflicted property damage exceeding 50 billion dollars. Half of the people affected by disasters are children. Over 18 million children were affected annually by disasters during the last five years alone. Unfortunately, we see no signs of these numbers diminishing. The severe impact of disasters on humanity becomes only more apparent as their frequency rises. In the past, the impact of war and conflict on humanity was measured by counting military casualties. This yardstick is no longer adequate. Victims in disasters are 5:1 civilian over military with the majority being women, children and the elderly. In 2013, as this manual is being revised, there are 2.2 million Syrian refugees distributed in several countries, 1.6 million Afghan refugees in Pakistan, 565,000 Somali refugees in Kenya, and more than 29 million people displaced within their own countries as a result of natural or man-made disasters. Every week there is at least one large crisis somewhere in the world that requires external assistance.

Overall mortality associated with disasters

Bosnia	250,000	people
Sudan	600,000	people
Rwanda	1,000,000	people
Tsunami	280,000	people
Haiti earthquake	159,000	people

EARLY AND LATE PHASES

Humanitarian work requires a broad perspective in order to effectively address the issues created by disasters. Disasters can be thought of in terms of distinct stages, frequently referred to as emergency and late phases.

- Early / Acute / Emergency phase

  - (0–1 month)

- Late / Recovery phase

  - (1–6 months)

- Rehabilitation / Development phase

  - (6+ months)

During the emergency phase of a disaster, the most urgent survival needs of the displaced persons must be met. Sometimes attention to the most urgent survival needs may be delayed by security issues. Once the situation is adequately secure, the most urgent needs to be addressed include food, water, sanitation, emergency shelter, health care and preliminary steps toward reunification. From the onset, relief efforts must be provided in a manner that ensures fair distribution. One of the most critical aspects of the emergency phase is to initiate record keeping with placement of identification bands, especially for children. It is in the chaos of the emergency phase that many children are separated from their families.

EMERGENCY PHASE RELIEF MEASURES

- **Triage:** both medical and psychological triage should be instituted immediately to Identify those most in need of help.

- **Immediate record-keeping:** name, age and gender of all incoming refugees or displaced persons, identification bands for children less than 10 years of age.

- **Rapid assessment of the emergency situation and the affected population:** define the magnitude, environmental conditions, major health/nutrition needs and local response capacity.

- **Provide adequate shelter and clothing:** exposure to elements can lead to death and increased caloric needs.

- **Provide adequate food:** ensure adequate calories and frequent meals for children, support breastfeeding.

- **Provide elementary sanitation and clean water:** minimum 3–6 L/person/day of reasonably clean water.

- **Institute diarrhea control program:** community education, improve sanitation and water source.

- **Immunize against measles and provide Vitamin A supplements:** Vitamin A decreases the fatality rate of measles.

- **Establish primary care medical treatment:** appropriate to the prevalent diseases and treatment standards of the local population.

- **Establish disease surveillance and a health information system:** monitor treatment effectiveness, realign priorities.

- **Organize human resources:** identify leaders for water and food distribution, community health workers, surrogate parents for unaccompanied minors.

- **Coordinate activities:** local authorities, relief organizations, military personnel.

Once the late phase of a disaster begins, it is appropriate to address a much broader field of concerns; the goals should expand on emergency phase issues and incorporate long-term needs. For example, late phase efforts should include the establishment of an expanded immunization program, maternal and child health programs, programs to address psychological problems, and educational systems for children and adults. Throughout a disaster, decisions must reflect the phase and needs of each situation.

ACUTE AND LONG-TERM EFFECTS

While it is common to describe the impact of disasters in terms of mortality, the associated morbidity is usually far worse. Morbidity is more challenging to measure. It may present as acute illness or injury, or as a myriad of serious, chronic problems. For decades after a disaster, the children and the world community continue to feel its chronic impact. The true depth and breadth of the long-term morbidity inflicted by disasters is frequently underestimated.

- **Mortality**: number of deaths.

- **Morbidity**: number of cases of illness or injury.

The acute causes of morbidity associated with disasters include an array of medical conditions. The most commonly encountered are diarrheal diseases, dehydration, respiratory illness, malaria, burns, trauma, fatigue/heat exhaustion and obstetric/neonatal emergencies. Although these may seem similar to the pathology found in adults, each of these conditions requires consideration of issues that are unique and critical to the care of children. Studies show that both children and adults experience immunosuppression during disasters; this may make them more susceptible to infectious diseases.

For example, while the nutrition of children is usually considered an acute issue, it can have lifelong consequences. A single episode of severe malnutrition during the first year of life has been associated with irreversible cognitive impairment. In addition, evidence from several studies suggests a causal relationship between under nutrition and behavioral development. We do not know to what extent the long-term outcomes of early malnutrition are negatively impacting the lives of millions of adults and the communities in which they live.

The psychological trauma inflicted upon children is one of the most difficult morbidities to appreciate in early phases of a disaster. Many studies demonstrate that disaster situations cause psychological trauma in children. It is now well accepted that man-made disasters are associated with a higher incidence of long-term psychological dysfunction than are natural disasters. The experience of psychological trauma varies depending on the age, developmental stage, and personality of the child. While the earliest signs of trauma may manifest during and immediately after a disaster, some children may manifest psychological problems years later. In some cases, children may never recover completely.

5. Natural Disasters and Children

Natural disasters include earthquakes, hurricanes or cyclones, floods, tsunamis, tornadoes, eruption of volcanoes, mudslides, and fires. Earthquakes are the least predictable. With good weather forecasting and media access, families in the path of some natural disasters such as hurricanes or floods may have time to escape. Families may escape injury or death from a tornado by moving to a basement area. In spite of escaping injury or death, families are likely to face loss of homes, property, and livelihoods. Children suffer both acutely and long term.

Hurricanes are tropical storms with winds at least 74 miles per hour (mph) with gusts sustained for at least one minute. The winds blow in a large spiral around a relatively calm center known as "The Eye" which may be 20–30 miles wide. The hurricane can extend 400 miles beyond the eye. Tropical Cyclones or Typhoons or Severe Tropical Cyclones are the terms used for Hurricanes in the southern hemisphere. A category 1 hurricane has winds up to 95 miles per hour. A category 2 hurricane is up to 110 mph. Extensive damage is caused by a category 3 (110–130 mph). Extreme damage occurs in a category 4 hurricane (131–155 mph) and a catastrophe when there is a category 5 hurricane with winds more than 155 mph. A storm surge is an onshore rush of ocean or lake water caused by high winds when the hurricane hits land. A hurricane storm tide is the surge plus the normal incoming tide in combination.

Floods are the most common natural disaster. Flash floods which occur during sudden heavy rains or when dams or levees give way are most hazardous. As little as two feet of rushing water can carry a vehicle away. Floodwaters are usually contaminated with sewage or chemicals. Areas covered by floodwaters are a hazard for long periods after the water has receded. Floods may also drive wild animals, including snakes, into areas where they are not usually found e.g. front yards of homes.

Tsunamis occur when underwater earthquakes result in the formation of gigantic waves that cross thousands of miles of ocean with speeds up to 500 miles an hour. They may crest at heights of 100 feet and may destroy buildings and cause deaths for several miles inland.

Earthquakes are a potential hazard in many areas of the world. Earthquake severity is measured in Richter units. Each increase in a Richter unit represents an increase in energy up to the highest level, number 8. On average two earthquakes of magnitude 8 occur each year and there are 20 earthquakes of a magnitude 7.

Fires include those within cities and in forest areas. They cause deaths, property damage, burns, and displacement of families.

Tornadoes are rotating masses of air which measure a few hundred meters across and usually travel over only a few miles of land. They can have winds up to 200 miles per hour. They may destroy entire small towns or large sections of cities.

Mudslides and eruption of volcanoes may cause huge destruction of communities. Although they are usually predictable and it is often possible for families to escape, the tragedy of complete destruction of homes and property will cause long-term displacement of children and their families.

All of these types of natural disasters have the potential to cause displacement of children and their families, causing the same types of problems as man-made disasters. Children may experience the death of their parents or family members.

Children may be separated from family members in the mad rush to safety, as occurred in the Asia tsunami of December 2004 and the Katrina hurricane related floods in 2005. They may experience acute fear from the sound of the tornado or hurricane or sight of debris flying or fires or rushing floodwaters.

They experience disruption of their usual life, often losing their familiar home and routines. Children may become ill from exposure to contaminated items such as toys found lying in the wake of a flood. They may be injured by debris or chemicals discovered while exploring in the aftermath of a disaster. Several studies have shown that many children experience symptoms of anxiety and fear for years after the experience of a natural disaster.

How can families and relief workers reduce the likelihood that children will experience physical or mental trauma in the wake of a natural disaster?

Most important is that families anticipate disasters when possible, plan an evacuation route and have disaster supplies on hand. These include flashlights with extra batteries, battery operated radios with extra batteries, first aid kits, emergency food and water, essential medications, cash, sturdy shoes, and an emergency communication plan with family members or friends in the event of a natural disaster. The fact that families plan and appear able to cope in the presence of a disaster is reassuring to their children.

Children who have survived a natural disaster and are displaced should be provided water, shelter, food, and medical care. Efforts should be made to establish routines for children in the wake of a natural disaster as soon as possible. School activities should be organized as soon as possible. Relief workers should help parents or guardians to recognize symptoms of anxiety or depression in children and to provide opportunities for them to ask questions or talk about the disaster if they wish. Provision of paper, crayons, modeling clay may be helpful to children who benefit by drawing or modeling what they have perceived in the disaster. Organized programs such as the UNICEF "Return to Happiness" (See Chapter 16 on Child Development) may be beneficial to children who have lived through a major disaster. Most of all, assistance to parents in reconstruction of their homes and lives will be of most benefit to their children.

6. The Major Players in Disaster Management

Throughout history, nations have responded to disaster situations by offering their own resources in aid as a "good neighbor gesture." As the number of disasters has risen over the past three decades, the need for external assistance has grown. In 1985, 22 million people were internally displaced or refugees; in 2012 this figure increased to 45.2 million people. These included 15.4 million refugees, 28.8 internally displaced people, and 937,000 asylum seekers. Over the years, a complex system of international humanitarian response has developed that involves governmental and non-governmental organizations (NGOs). The major players in this system are listed here and are then described in more detail below.

The United Nations (UN)

- UN Office for Coordination of Humanitarian Affairs (OCHA)

- UN High Commissioner for Refugees (UNHCR)

- World Food Program (WFP)

- World Health Organization (WHO)

- The United Nations Children's Fund (UNICEF)

- Inter Agency Standing Committee (IASC)

International Red Cross and Red Crescent Movement

- International Committee of the Red Cross (ICRC)

- International Federation of Red Cross and Red Crescent Societies

- National Red Cross and Red Crescent Societies
  Office of United States Foreign Disaster Assistance

Coalition Military

- Civil-Military Operations Center (COMC)

- Peacekeeping and Peace Enforcement

Local Government Organizations

- Ministries of Health

- District Health Directors

Non-Governmental Organizations (NGOs), selected examples

- American Refugee Committee (ARC)

- Cooperative for American Relief Everywhere (CARE)

- Catholic Relief Services (CRS)

- International Rescue Committee (IRC)

- Medicins Sans Frontiers (MSF) / Doctors Without Borders

- Oxford Committee for Famine Relief (OXFAM)

- Save the Children Fund

- World Vision

The Sphere Project

THE UNITED NATIONS AGENCIES

The United Nations (UN) was established in 1945 as the administrative body of a multilateral treaty, which is voluntarily endorsed by supporting nations. According to its 1948 charter, the UN is charged with safeguarding human rights and equal rights for all nations. The UN involvement in international situations is limited by the conditions of its multilateral treaty. Specifically, the UN cannot impose "the threat or use of force against the territorial integrity or political independence of any state." In addition, it cannot provide aid across uninvited borders. This latter provision can be over-ridden by the Security Council, which is a smaller governing body of leading nations within the UN. If international security is threatened, the UN Security Council can dismiss the national sovereignty policies. However, the time restraints inherent to this process lead to significant delays in the UN response to many disasters.

OCHA (formerly Department of Humanitarian Affairs)

The OCHA coordinates humanitarian assistance for the UN. The OCHA advises the UN Secretary-General regarding emergency situations, oversees the coordination of UN agencies in response to disasters and mobilizes the international community. In emergency situations, the OCHA unifies the various UN relief agencies and coordinates their efforts with non-UN organizations, principally NGOs. Theoretically, the OCHA has the ability to mobilize funds quickly. It can then direct this funding to non-UN organizations, since these non-UN organizations are often able to respond more quickly in an emergency situation.

The UNHCR

The United Nations High Commissioner for Refugees (UNHCR) was established by the United Nations General Assembly in 1951. Prior to 1990, the UNHCR mandate was to guarantee the protection of refugee populations and to find permanent solutions to their situations. Since then it has been expanded to include action to prevent refugee movements. Based on this expanded mandate, the UNHCR can provide assistance to civilian populations who are victims of hostilities, regardless of refugee status. Thus, the UNHCR may provide assistance to populations who are not externally displaced.

The IASC

The Inter Agency Standing Committee is the primary mechanism for inter-agency coordination of humanitarian assistance. It is a forum involving key UN and non-UN humanitarian partners. It was established in 1992.

The WFP

The World Food Program (WFP) was created in 1961 to provide food aid to non-industrialized countries. This aid is offered in the form of economic development programs and emergency relief. The WFP is designed to target food towards special segments of the population, such as children, lactating women and the elderly. The WFP also coordinates efforts with other UN agencies and with local NGOs. For example, the WFP may coordinate with the local Red Cross group, such that the local group takes responsibility for food distribution.

The WHO

From the beginning, the UN acknowledged the critical need for improving the health of humanity. This is evident in a memorable quote from the 1945 discussions: "Medicine *is one of the pillars of peace*" (US Archbishop, later Cardinal Spellman). To this end, the World Health Organization (WHO) was established in 1946 to act as a directing and coordinating authority in international health. The WHO gives assistance to governments on request.

In June 1948, the First World Health Assembly convened to determine the priorities of the WHO. Although its main focus was disease control, it also emphasized the socioeconomic, cultural and political dimensions of health. The first two decades of WHO were dominated by campaigns against malaria, tuberculosis, small pox, yaws, syphilis and leprosy, among many other diseases.

The UNICEF

The United Nations Children's Fund (UNICEF), created in 1946, is mandated to protect children and to promote the application of the Convention on the Rights of the Child around the world. The convention specifies that children have the right to enjoy the best health possible. UNICEF's field activities are diverse; they address nutrition, water supply, immunizations, education, material provision, management, logistics and technical support to social programs. The general assembly created UNICEF as an organization to provide assistance to all countries worldwide. Although most of its activities fall into the area of development, UNICEF does intervene in emergency situations. Unlike other UN agencies, UNICEF may provide assistance even without permission of existing governments. Also, UNICEF may raise funds from private sources. All other UN agencies rely on monies donated from member nations.

THE INTERNATIONAL RED CROSS AND RED CRESCENT MOVEMENT

The International Red Cross and Red Crescent Movement encompass the International Committee of the Red Cross (ICRC), the International Federation of the Red Cross and Red Crescent Societies and all of the recognized National Red Cross and Red Crescent Societies. The Federation serves as the central secretariat of the National Red Cross and Red Crescent Societies. In 1989, an agreement was made between the ICRC and the Federation that clearly delineates the roles and responsibilities of each individual organization. The ICRC heads the Movement's international activities in armed conflicts and other situations requiring a specifically neutral and independent organization. The Federation Coordinates the National Societies efforts in peacetime and disaster situations.

The highest deliberating body of the Movement is the International Conference of the Red Cross and Red Crescent. This body promotes dialogue with the signatory States of the Geneva Convention and provides a forum in which States can be brought to confront the responsibilities this law imposes on them. The International Conference can pass resolutions, make recommendations and formulate draft proposals concerning international humanitarian conventions. In addition, it can assign mandates to the ICRC and the Federation.

The ICRC

The ICRC is the world's oldest relief organization. It was founded in 1863 as the International Committee for Relief to Soldiers, adopting the symbol of a red cross on a white background. In the following year, the Swiss Federal Council organized an international conference, where the Geneva Convention for the Amelioration of the Condition of the Wounded in Armies in the Field was created. In 1880, the International Committee for the Relief of Soldiers officially adopted the name of the International Committee of the Red Cross.

Through the Geneva Conventions and their additional protocols, the international community has placed mandates on the ICRC. In 1977, protocols were added to the Conventions that specifically address internal and international conflict/civil disturbances (such as disasters).

As described in article nine of the Geneva Convention, the ICRC has the right and the duty to intercede across borders in both international and non-international conflicts. This mandate supersedes any existing government. When there is no identifiable protecting power, as is the situation in many disasters, the ICRC serves to safeguard the interests and humanitarian functional needs of the victims. In 1990, the United Nations General Assembly granted the ICRC observer status.

The role of the ICRC includes maintaining and disseminating the Fundamental Principles of the Movement, namely humanity, impartiality, neutrality, independence, voluntary service, unity and universality (Article 4). By functioning as a neutral, independent humanitarian provider, the ICRC offers relief assistance and legal protection to victims.

The neutrality of the ICRC is essential to its role in any relief operation. In the case of disasters, the ICRC will be present only if the parties in conflict agree to recognize and uphold the ICRC's neutrality. The ICRC offers assistance to people regardless of their nationality, color, religion, social position or political affiliations. The details of every ICRC relief convoy are completely disclosed to all belligerent parties. By operating on all sides of the conflict, the ICRC ensures its neutrality.

The International Federation of Red Cross and Red Crescent Societies

The Federation was founded in 1919, during the aftermath of World War I. Its general objective is "to inspire, encourage, facilitate and promote at all times all forms of humanitarian activities by the National Societies with a view to preventing and alleviating human suffering and thereby contributing to the maintenance and the promotion of peace in the world." It also serves to organize, coordinate and direct international relief actions and represent the National Societies at the international level.

In 1994, the International Red Cross and Red Crescent Movement joined with six of the world's oldest and largest NGOs to outline a professional Code of Conduct. This describes the universal basic standards by which the Movement and registered NGOs should work in disaster assistance. The ten principal points by which signatories have voluntarily agreed to abide are:

- The humanitarian imperative comes first.

- Aid is given regardless of race, creed or nationality of the recipients and without adverse distinction of any kind. Aid priorities are calculated on the basis of need alone.

- Aid will not be used to further a particular political or religious standard.

- We shall endeavor not to act as instruments of government foreign policy.

- We shall respect culture and custom.

- We shall attempt to build disaster response on local capabilities.

- Ways shall be found to involve program beneficiaries in the management of relief aid.

- Relief aid must strive to reduce future vulnerabilities to disaster, as well as meeting basic needs.

- We hold ourselves accountable to both those we seek to assist and those from whom we accept resources.

- In our information, publicity and advertising activities, we shall recognize disaster victims as dignified humans, not hopeless objects.

The National Red Cross and Red Crescent Societies

The National Societies have roles in both peacetime and armed conflict. In peacetime, the National Societies' activities are generally concentrated in areas of health, health education and natural-disaster relief. With support from the Federation, the National Societies work in areas as diverse as blood donation, disease and epidemic prevention, first aid, social welfare, AIDS prevention and treatment, communication systems and disaster-preparedness programs. When called upon by the ICRC, the National societies offer relief assistance to the victims of armed conflicts. The ICRC may call upon health care personnel from countries that are not involved in the conflict.

OFFICE OF THE UNITED STATES FOREIGN DISASTER ASSISTANCE (OFDA)

This office is part of USAID and is divided into three divisions:

The Disaster Response and Mitigation (DRM) division is responsible for coordinating with other organizations for the provision of relief supplies and humanitarian assistance. The **Operations Division (OPS)** develops and manages logistical, operational, and technical support for disaster responses. OPS maintains readiness to respond to emergencies through several mechanisms, including managing several Search and Rescue (SAR) Teams, the Ground Operations Team (GO Team), field Disaster Assistance Response Teams (DART), and the Washington Response Management teams (RMT). The **Program Support (PS)** division provides programmatic and administrative support.

NON-GOVERNMENTAL ORGANIZATIONS (NGOs)

Although NGOs number more than 20,000 worldwide, only a small percentage of these are involved in disaster and humanitarian relief. About 30 NGOs provide 95% of the assistance in disasters. Most NGOs are small, originate in industrialized nations and focus on development projects. Since their perspective is affected by individual strengths, NGOs usually find a niche of needs that they target.

NGOs base their actions on the principle that the rights of suffering people transcend the principles of sovereignty and non-interference. Unlike the ICRC, NGOs have engaged in cross-border operations without the approval of the host government. In addition, not all NGOs maintain a position of neutrality. Some NGOs have spoken out openly against the atrocities of individual governments. Consequently, NGOs may risk provoking hostility from warring factions.

In disasters, NGOs share the common goal of relieving misery from disease and starvation. However, as a relief system they tend to function in a loose framework. They vary in size, structure, objectives, religious and non-religious affiliations. The NGOs ability to succeed in their task is largely based on their ability to mobilize funds. Thus, all NGOs compete with each other for a limited allocation of resources. In many cases, NGOs receive funding from UN agencies. The NGOs then work in coordination with the UN agencies as implementing partners.

NGOs may also receive funding through grants from governments. In the case of US foreign aid, the source of funding is the United States Agency for International Development (USAID). In emergency situations, the Office of Foreign Disaster Assistance (OFDA) and their Disaster Assessment Response Team (DART) coordinate disaster response in the field. Ideally, this arrangement provides the most expeditious allocation of funds. Defined by law, OFDA may assist in providing basic needs (food, water, shelter, sanitation, medical care and heat). Thus, OFDA is not involved in the provision of funds for development and/or reconstruction.

Over the past 30 years NGOs have emerged as the agencies primarily responsible for providing assistance to those in need during disasters. In recent years, the environment of disasters has become more ambiguous and tense with worsening security. Despite increasing danger, NGOs persist in their efforts to provide humanitarian aid. Greater emphasis is being placed on the preparation and training of NGO workers. It is critical that NGO workers be proficient in basic self-preservation and security behaviors. NGO workers must also be aware of land mine locations and public health indicators. Finally, NGO workers must fully comprehend the interactions between tribal, clan and/or warring factions; recognize who to work with among local leaders; and learn how to collaborate respectfully with those leaders, without causing offense.

COALITION MILITARY FORCES

During emergency situations, security is provided by the UN in the form of peacekeeping or peace-enforcing military forces. Sanctioned by the Security Council, member nations must contribute military units to a coalition force. The utilization of a coalition force sanctioned by the UN Security Council was established by the precedent set during the Kurdish refugee crisis in 1991. Due to the essential nature of establishing the security of relief operations, the coalition military and the UN humanitarian agencies/DHA are operationally in charge of these military forces.

The Kurdish refugee crisis is recognized as being the first occasion during which NGOs and the military were able to create an effective collaborative relationship. By perceiving the military as an ally, NGOs were able to accomplish their humanitarian activities through use of the coalition's protective transport, communication and shelter. The success of the Kurdish crisis is frequently attributed to the military's fielding of an unusually high number of personnel drawn from the civil affairs units. These personnel, competent in civil administration, medicine and engineering, complemented the NGO community well. Military resources were also made available to NGOs involved in the Rwandan humanitarian crisis in 1994. Military groups from several countries were based in Goma and took responsibility for water purification, immunizations, and mobile hospitals.

The role of the military is limited to the emergency phase of disasters only. All military troops may have duties that include true humanitarian service roles. Under UN Chapter VI, peacekeeping actions can include defensive military operations to monitor an existing agreement between warring factions, and are undertaken only with the consent of all belligerent parties. The troops are supplied for primarily non-combat roles. In chapter VII, peace-enforcing actions are provided to compel compliance with UN Security Council resolutions. These interventions involve armed military forces.

LOCAL GOVERNMENT ORGANIZATIONS

Working in collaboration with local government organizations is essential to the success of any disaster endeavor, large or small. In some unfortunate situations, there may be no effective local government. In all other situations, the local government organizations should be involved as soon as possible. Local governments provide unique insights into disaster situations. Including the local government in initial assessment and planning efforts can expedite processes and provide the local community with a sense of ownership.

THE SPHERE PROJECT

The Sphere Project, begun in 1997, is a voluntary initiative that brings a wide range of humanitarian agencies together around a common aim—to improve the quality of humanitarian assistance and the accountability of humanitarian actors to the affected populations, constituents and donors. The Sphere Project is guided by a board with 18 members who represent a global network of humanitarian agencies. Its office is hosted by the International Federation of the Red Cross and Red Crescent in Geneva, Switzerland. The Sphere Project Handbook, *Humanitarian Charter and Minimum Standards in Disaster Response*, is widely known and was updated in 2011.

THE CLUSTER APPROACH

The Cluster Approach was initiated as part of a UN Humanitarian Reform process. It was first tried immediately after the 2005 earthquake in Pakistan where nine clusters were established within 24 hours. The purpose of the Cluster Approach is to enhance partnerships and complementarity among the UN, Red Cross and NGO agencies, and to use available resources efficiently.

At a country level clusters will normally be established for any major emergency in areas such as health, water and sanitation, protection, shelter, food and education. The clusters are established according to the varying needs of every disaster situation and also according to which relief agencies are available in a given disaster. They are designated by the Inter Agency Standing Committee (IASC). OCHA established a Humanitarian Coordinating Support Section (HCSS) which is based in Geneva to support Humanitarian Coordinators in disaster areas and also the IASC partners.

SUMMARY

Although the disaster response system has evolved to serve and protect the most vulnerable in emergency situations, it is extremely complex. It is a system that is both difficult to understand and within which to work. Relief workers should pay attention to which agencies are present in each disaster situation, to what resources each agency has, and who is in charge. They must also determine what reporting responsibilities they have. In the midst of policy-making and mandate enforcement, the children are frequently forgotten. It is important to include the needs of children in planning.. With respect to each decision, it is useful to ask the questions, "How does this affect the children and their future? What is best for children?

7. Priorities for Children

Children require special attention in disasters. A careful, proactive approach from the start can make a remarkable difference in outcomes for children affected by disasters. Children are not miniature versions of adults; they have unique needs that make them particularly vulnerable during disasters. Unlike adults, children lack the reserves required to endure acute stress. Due to their small size and different metabolic function, they develop dehydration, malnutrition and fatigue more quickly. Hence, the provision of water, appropriate food, a place to rest, and a clean environment must occur more rapidly for children than for adults.

Children are also different in their susceptibility to illness and psychological stress. For example, children have immature immune systems and are more likely to contract infectious diseases than adults. In addition, these diseases tend to be more severe in children. Disasters also cause disruption in critical stages of child development. Many children experience separation from adult caretakers. While separation from support systems is known to be associated with poor health outcomes in all people, this is particularly true for unaccompanied minors who have lost parental protection. The ability to process trauma and loss is made more difficult by the fact that most children do not think abstractly until age 16 or later. This is an important consideration in addressing the mental health needs of children who experience disasters.

The basic requirements of children involved in disasters include food, clothing, shelter and sanitation. Although these appear no different from those of adults, their successful provision to children requires different considerations. Ensuring fair and effective distribution of supplies to children is one of the greatest challenges facing relief workers.

FOOD

For infants, food is breast milk. Substitutes are only considered acceptable in extreme situations. The supply of breast milk is sensitive to many factors, including maternal stress, hydration, physiology, nutrition and birth spacing. It is therefore critical that lactating women be given supplemental nutrition and psychological support. If breastfeeding mothers do not have milk, efforts must be made to find wet nurses or suitable formula which can be prepared in a sanitary manner.

For children, the fact that they have smaller total caloric requirements than adults does not simplify the situation. Children need smaller, more frequent portions of food. If young children are given their entire ration of food in one sitting, adults or older children who can tolerate larger portions will ultimately eat the food. This leads to total caloric deprivation of younger children. In addition, children are more sensitive to micronutrient deficiencies than adults.

Of particular importance is fair distribution of the food supply. Children are usually dependent on adults for their supply of resources. In situations where adults are not present or reliable, relief workers must assume the role of provider and protector. For instance, one way to ensure fair distribution of the food supply is to create separate areas for providing meals to children.

CLOTHING

The issue of children's clothing is frequently overlooked, despite being a basic need. In warm, resource poor areas, children may often play barefooted and wear little clothing. This is not acceptable attire in an unnatural, stressful situation such as a disaster. Being naked and barefoot in a disaster leads to unjustified suffering for children and places them at increased risk for infectious disease and trauma. Providing children with clothing that fits their size will help lessen the likelihood that the clothing will be taken from them by older children or adults.

SHELTER AND PROTECTION

For children, shelter not only incorporates protection from the elements, but also protection from exploitation, abuse and negative influences of some adults. Unfortunately, children are the easiest targets for corrupt adults in disaster settings. When children are exposed to negative influences and poor adult role modeling, the negative effects can be long lasting.

Many children affected by disasters are in the midst of critical phases of development with respect to a sense of values. For example, children aged seven to twelve years are learning to formulate concepts of right and wrong (concrete operations). During puberty, children begin to perform abstract thought processes (formal operations), which include exploration of morality issues.

When children lack appropriate role models during these developmental stages, the end result can be devastating; children may be develop a warped sense of values. This outcome can have a devastating effect on the communities where these children live as adults. Examples include situations in which young children are forced to become soldiers of war, perform brutal acts of violence, murder/ maim their own family members or are subject to sexual abuse and rape.

In many disaster situations, creating separate facilities for children may be the safest solution. During the emergency phase, it is essential to identify and collectively house all unaccompanied minors. Gender differences should be considered in arranging shelter for older children. Eventually, foster care arrangements should be made for all unaccompanied minors. During the late phase of disasters, it is important to create areas where routine, safe group activities can take place for children under supervision of responsible adults.

Housing arrangements for children must take into account safe access to latrines. Adults should accompany young children to latrines, and older children should not go to latrines alone when it is dark.

SANITATION

Children prove to be a particular challenge in the area of sanitation. Children find it natural to defecate and urinate indiscreetly. For this reason, children are the most difficult group in which to create compliance in the use of defecation fields, latrines and basic hygiene. Not only are children more likely to be victims of infectious disease, but they are also prime spreaders of infectious diseases. Efforts to educate children and provide adult role models in the area of sanitation will have a great impact on the incidence of infectious disease spread by the fecal-oral route.

THE IMPORTANCE OF ESTABLISHING ROUTINES FOR CHILDREN

Resilience in children who experience a disaster is facilitated by routines. These provide some predictability and regularity which is comforting to children. Attention to routines includes regular timing of meals, a defined place for sleeping, regular play times, the same caretakers, and re-establishment of schools.

HEALTH CARE

The delivery of pediatric medical care must be adapted to the age and stage of child patients. Clinicians should take care to approach children in a child-friendly manner. Since young children frequently cannot express or describe their symptoms, health care workers must be sensitive to body language and physical cues. To successfully observe and gather this information, health care workers must make special efforts to create a non-threatening and comfortable examination environment.

A comforting approach for younger children is to ask a mother to undress her child and to keep the child seated on her lap. Keeping easily cleaned toys as distractors in the clinic area is also helpful The clinician can then complete the history while observing the child seated comfortably with the mother. An experienced child health care provider can acquire a majority of the diagnostic information prior to physically touching the child. For example, when undressed and comfortably seated in the mother's arms, a child in respiratory distress can be clearly identified by visual examination. If this same child is frightened and crying throughout the physical exam, it may be difficult to collect useful information.

Children have many specific medical issues that are either unique to them or have different presentations than in adults. These will be discussed in greater detail in later chapters; two examples are presented here:

Dehydration: The consequences of dehydration are often more severe in children. For example, adults infected with rotavirus may experience several days of fever, diarrhea and discomfort. For infants, this infection can be fatal. Infants and children become dehydrated much more rapidly than adults. Some factors that contribute to this are a lack of stored excess body fluids and the increased loss of body fluids that children experience due to their increased body surface to body mass ratio. In addition, infants under seven months of age are at greater risk of electrolyte abnormalities due to the diminished concentrating ability of their kidneys. These electrolyte abnormalities can lead to severe complications from dehydration, These include seizures, cardiac arrhythmia, stroke and loss of limbs.

Medications: Children require special consideration in the use of medications. Medication doses need to be calculated on the basis of weight in children. They may be absorbed or metabolized differently in children who are malnourished or in children who are also receiving indigenous oral treatments such as herbs. Children experience different side effects than adults and possess varying abilities to swallow oral medications. Their compliance with medical advice is generally dependent on adults.

These examples illustrate how helpful it can be to have child health specialists present in disasters. However, all relief workers need to have a basic understanding of the special needs of children in order to provide them effective services.

8.   Unaccompanied Minors

The separation of children from their parents has serious, far-reaching consequences. Parents are the main providers for all children. Without them, children suffer from lost access to resources and emotional insecurity. Children who are separated from their parents or adult caretakers in disasters are called unaccompanied minors. These children may have become separated during the initial exodus from their family home; they may have become lost in a crowd; they may have been abandoned; their family members may have died. It is frightening and traumatic for children to lose their parents anytime and especially during a disaster.

During the initial period of separation, unaccompanied minors suffer from a loss of all basic requirements, leaving them at high risk for malnutrition, infectious disease and exploitation. Due to their lack of experience and their inability to think abstractly, children are at a disadvantage without the guidance of adults. It is critical that children be provided with a safe, supportive and stable environment. Loss of such an environment during childhood can cause serious developmental and psychological trauma that can affect children for a lifetime.

EMERGENCY PHASE

Humanitarian workers must take a proactive approach to the issue of unaccompanied minors. It is clear from previous disasters that children are at high risk for separation from their parents or adult caretakers during population movements. Although difficult to obtain in statistical form, the numbers affected are large. Many of these separations can be prevented if an identification or record keeping system is quickly established for children and families entering a camp. Once separation has occurred, a few basic principles can guide humanitarian workers and lessen the traumatic impact on children.

- **Have an established plan.** Prepare yourself and fellow workers; assess the setting and resources; establish a plan for unaccompanied minors.

- **Take a proactive approach.** Prevent the separation of children from adult caretakers. Give adults mechanisms to help keep track of their children. For example, family identification cards can be pinned on children's shirts or can be worn as tags or wristbands.

- **Attempt immediate reunification.** When an unaccompanied minor is identified, immediately try to find an adult nearby who knows the child. A relative or neighbor who will take responsibility for the child is the best alternative if the parent cannot be found. This gives the child the best chance of returning to his/her family.

- **Document immediately.** Record information about the separated child in as much detail as possible. Write down whatever the child or other witnesses tell you. Take pictures of the child before bathing or changing his/her clothes. This is especially important for toddlers who cannot identify themselves.

- **Find foster homes and surrogate caregivers.** In general children do better in foster situations than in orphanages. Orphanages are generally not a good replacement for family and community living. The SOS orphanage program is an exception which exists in many countries, guarantees loving support to orphans through higher education, and raises children in a pleasant home with 7 or 8 other children. It is important to be aware of different norms and expectations regarding foster care and adoption in different cultural settings.

- **Discourage the misconception that "children are better off with the relief workers."** Mothers have been known to pretend that their children are unaccompanied minors in order to place them in the care of relief workers in hopes that the children will have better access to resources.

LATE PHASE

During the later phases of disasters, the specific needs of children continue to differ from those of adults. An overriding theme is that children require a safe, stable environment in which to grow—an environment that gives them a sense of physical and emotional security. The creation of a sense of community, with provision of surrogate parents for unaccompanied minors, is essential to foster normal growth and development. In addition, children must be protected against exposure to harmful experiences. All unaccompanied minors have undoubtedly survived traumatic experiences. Special care must be taken to shield them from additional insults.

Once again, humanitarian workers must provide for basic needs in a child-friendly manner. In addition, they must take the responsibility of safe guarding the children's portions of food, shelter and clothes. Basic medical care designed for children is essential, beginning with a thorough assessment of the children's medical conditions, immunization coverage and nutritional status. All medical programs should include an appropriate program of immunizations, careful growth and nutritional monitoring, supplemental feeding programs and psychological assessments.

Children do suffer from the long-term consequences of psychological trauma. Frequently, they show symptoms of such trauma in ways that are not obvious to adults. For example, children may regress developmentally; they may have frequent nightmares; they may be hyperactive or inattentive; they may become aggressive or withdrawn; they may engage in repetitive behaviors. Continual surveillance for these symptoms and others is necessary. Provision of paper and pens and crayons may encourage children to draw. Often the drawings reveal a great deal about their fears and concerns. Ideally, child health specialists should be present in all disasters to provide preventive and therapeutic counseling for children. At a minimum, humanitarian workers should provide children with culturally appropriate avenues in which to express themselves in their everyday lives. This is the first step to a healthy recovery.

It is important that humanitarian workers foster and nurture a sense of hope for the future in children affected by disasters. It has been demonstrated that hopelessness is associated with an increased risk of death. A practical and useful method of instilling hope is through education. When people start learning, they begin to live for the future. For small children, school offers a normal, structured routine that they desperately need. Adolescents benefit from school in many ways; it gives them a sense of purpose and bolsters their concept of personal identity. In addition, caretakers can be incorporated into the educational process. This is an excellent opportunity to make an impact on child health and child care behaviors.

9.   Priorities for Women

Nancy A. Hazleton

Women and children represent 75 percent of the population in many complex humanitarian emergencies and disasters. With the publication of the UNHCR Guidelines for Refugee Women, these specialized needs have at last become recognized and codified in policy documents. However, policy only presents a first step. In order for these guidelines to become a reality, implementation is of critical importance. As women represent caregivers and, in many instances, have become the heads of families, their roles are in flux. Important considerations in planning stable living situations for them are:

PHYSICAL SAFETY

Women's physical safety should be foremost in the minds of camp designers and administrators. There have been many reports of how women were physically in danger when engaging in daily living activities such as laundry and foraging for firewood. Attention must be given to how the risk of physical violence toward women can be eliminated.

HYGIENE AND PUBLIC HEALTH

Since women are the primary caregivers in the family unit, clean surroundings and water will not only help to ensure the health of the children under women's care, but also help to maintain the health of mothers. Basic public health measures of hygiene, clean and available water supplies, and waste disposal are essential. If possible, invest in the overall health of the family unit as a way of protecting the health of the individuals in that family. Often when a mother is ill, there is no one to care for her children and she is unable or unwilling to leave her living area for medical attention.

Women's special hygiene needs include sanitary supplies. Without this basic item available and provided, as a matter of course, to all women past puberty, women are unable to leave their living environment, to receive health care, cook, or receive food distributions.

Cotton cloths can be used and reused for this function. Areas should be made available where the cloths can be washed and hung out privately. This very important matter is often ignored in disaster situations.

Women's latrines and bathing areas should be kept separate from latrines for men. In these separate areas, space can be made for washing and drying sanitary supplies. In a CHE situation with its inherent personal loss and devastation, the recognition of personal dignity and privacy can be reassuring to women.

FOOD DISTRIBUTION

Since many women and children are separated from their husbands and fathers in a disaster, food distribution should not be given only to males. Efforts should be made either to take food to where the women are or to arrange for separate distribution schedules to the women. Prior to the initiation of transportation of any food supplies, dietary preferences should be studied and food familiar to the refugee group should then be sent. Consideration should be given to how women get fuel for cooking, other cooking supplies, and how to increase the ease of cooking for them.

SHELTER

The purpose of shelter is to provide protection from the elements, warmth and privacy. While imported materials can be used, it is preferable to use local building materials, if available. Providing these materials to women increases their sense of self-determination through building their own environment in a culturally familiar way. If local building materials are unavailable, it is preferable that housing be built in smaller scale clusters with latrines, food distribution centers, laundry and health care facilities in the immediate area. This can prevent the security and privacy problems that are frequent in large "tent cities."

HEALTH CARE

While a range of health care services are appropriate for all groups, such as immunizations and emergency care, the special health care needs of women must be recognized and planned for in a detailed manner. Reproductive health care (including prenatal, perinatal, and post-partum services) is essential in any health operation, but critical in disasters where there are more adult women than men. Gynecologic care with specialized attention to those women who have experienced genital mutilation and subsequent health problems should be available in private areas and provided by culturally sensitive staff. Many women feel more comfortable with female medical providers and this preference should be accommodated if possible.

Health visits provided at home are beneficial to mothers and children and can be accomplished through a system of indigenous health extenders who know the language and health customs of the women.

Midwives and doulas (labor and delivery companions) from the local culture may be enlisted to provide prenatal, delivery and postpartum services. WHO training manuals on normal labor and delivery are available for the education of midwives, doulas and other community health workers.

Women who have experienced sexual violence should be provided with appropriate physical and mental health services.

HIV/AIDS may be common in many disaster situations. Efforts to prevent transmission of HIV and other sexually transmitted illnesses (STIs) should include treatment of STIs, general health and sex education, distribution of condoms, family planning services, and linkages to local organizations that provide HIV prevention and/or treatment services. Of particular importance is provision of PMTCT (Prevention of Mother-To-Child Transmission) services to pregnant women.

Every culture has its own pharmacopoeia, healers and medical traditions that are familiar and comforting to its peoples. The WHO estimates that more than 60% of the world's population uses some form of traditional medicine. Enlisting traditional healers in disaster health plans may benefit the patient, family, and community. While efforts should be made to acknowledge and work with traditional healers, it is also important to be careful and not promote medications or practices that may be harmful or take unfair economic advantage of disaster victims.

POLICY-MAKING

An important way to ensure that the needs of women with respect to physical safety, hygiene, food distribution, shelter, and health care are met in disasters is to have experienced women on the planning and implementation teams. The common experiences of women as child-bearers, caretakers, homemakers and food preparers provide understanding that crosses cultural and geographic boundaries. Sensitivity to the special needs of women can lead to reductions in morbidity and mortality of both women and children. More women are needed to work in the international agency policy-making that drives relief efforts, as well as to work on the ground in disaster situations. The female victims of disasters should be involved in making plans related to health, social services and logistics that affect themselves and their families.

10. Triage and Children

Triage is an important concept for humanitarian workers when receiving training to work in disasters. The word "triage", from Old French trier, means to sort out. Triage involves sorting patients with the best chance of survival according to the available resources.

In large health emergencies the egalitarian approach, used daily by health professionals, is substituted by the utilitarian approach. Egalitarian could be defined as a belief in equal political, economic, social and civil rights for all people. Utilitarian approach is defined by some as the greater good for the greatest number of people. The utilitarian approach is used when the needs are greater than the available resources. As an example, in a disaster, if surgeons are not available a patient needing surgery is not treated and a patient, who does not require surgery, therefore having a better chance of survival according to the circumstances, is treated instead.

During the triage process only one person, the triage officer, should be in charge of making decisions. In emergencies, the decisions should be simple and clear to avoid confusion. It is very important to respect triage decisions.

There are different systems or tools, used to implement medical triage in Mass Casualty Incidents (MCI). The START (Simple Triage and Rapid Triage, 1983) and JumpSTART systems (Romig 1995) have been the most used tools. Both methods classify patients according to need for treatment and assign colors according to classification. They both classify different groups as follow: need for immediate care, (red), need for care that can be delayed (yellow), need for minimal or no care (green), and patients who are not expected to survive, or expectant death (black). JumpSTART is a system to triage children using physiologically appropriate decision points reflecting variations in normal children.

START and JumpSTART have been used for many years, but have not been validated. There is growing evidence favoring the ThinkSharp's Sacco Triage Method (STM). It is a scoring method in which victims are scored, and tagged. Victims are organized at the scene into three score groups, not color. Precision in scoring allows all responders to "speak the same language". Physiological scores are based on respiratory rate, pulse, motor response, with simple adjustment for age, and can be computed in about 40 seconds. The STM mathematical model incorporates outcome data from thousands of pediatric trauma patients, making it the only MCI triage tool for children that is based on data and is being clinically validated by objective means. The STM is used among all ages, but takes the special needs of children into consideration.

In children affected by disasters it is extremely important to assess, not only the physical injuries, but also the emotional and psychological trauma they have suffered. PsySTART (Schreiber 2005) assesses high risk and links high risk to short term evidence based interventions. Emerging evidence suggests some interventions can alter the risk and prevent PTSD (post-traumatic stress disorder). First responders can identify children who have had most traumatic experiences. Mental health practitioners then interview those children about perception of threat and subjective experience of fear.

Medical triage, which sorts individuals to maximize the number of lives saved, is different from public health triage. Public health triage is defined as the sorting or identifying of populations for priority interventions. An example is the need to implement public health triage in the event of a need for mass immunizations following exposures to meningitis, when there are insufficient doses of vaccine for everyone.

Humanitarian workers, independent of their specific areas of expertise, i.e. medical care, mental health services, or public health, need to familiarize themselves with the ethical overtones of triage under extreme circumstances in which the daily standards of care are altered.

11. Child Health Assessments

In the emergency phase of a disaster it is important to do the following assessments with respect to child health:

- "Eyeballing" the children as you walk through the area or as you observe children who may be walking by in refugee groups. Note how the children are dressed, whether or not they have shoes, how many of them appear dehydrated, their general state of nutrition, evidence of injuries, evidence of fear or anxiety and whether or not there appear to be unaccompanied minors. Are mothers able to breastfeed young infants?

- Do a survey of those children who are attending an acute care clinic or tent. What are the diagnoses? The most common problems? Do you find evidence of measles, malaria, meningitis, dysentery, dehydration and/or malnutrition? Keep careful records on the first 200–300 children you see. This information can provide a guide to acute prevention programs, needed supplies, drugs, and equipment, and for reporting to local authorities.

- If possible, get copies of immunization records (e.g. health passbooks) or oral reports with respect to immunization histories for a sample of children. This information can guide immunization programs, as well as help health workers anticipate the infectious diseases for which children are at risk.

- Develop an assessment of mortality via body counts or interviews with a specific number of families.

- Do a formal nutrition survey as soon as possible.

- Arrange for a survey related to potential post-traumatic stress problems. Arrange for interviews with a sample of families in order to learn which stressors have been most common for the children. These may include deaths of family members, witnessing violence, starvation, personal abuse, loss of home, cold weather and acute illness.

- The above sampling should also include an assessment of parental capacity. What stressors and privations have they endured? Are they malnourished? Are they ill or injured? Are the women pregnant? How many are breastfeeding? Are fathers present?

It is preferable to use sound epidemiological principles when doing such surveys. However, delaying these assessments and surveys because one lacks a measuring board or because the tents are moved frequently is not in the best interests of the children. Furthermore, it is important to survey and act on the information gained as soon as the survey results are known.

NUTRITIONAL ASSESSMENT

A nutrition survey is especially important when a majority of refugees are children under five years of age. The basic information to be collected includes:

- weight
- height
- age
- sex
- color of hair
- presence of edema

The plan for a nutritional survey should be developed in collaboration with displaced persons who are leaders. These leaders can help select people to assist in data collection. In general, one develops small teams that include two measurers and a supervisor. Before embarking on the formal survey, the team members should practice correct measurements; these must be checked.

Weight

In acute situations, the scale used for young children is usually a 25 kilogram (kg) hanging spring scale, graduated by 0.1 kg. The scale is hooked to a tree or to a stick held by two people. Although weighing pants are often used in Africa, many Asian villages have perfected the use of a comfortable weighing bamboo basket, which is much more acceptable to young children. In cold countries and in some cultures it may be impossible to undress a child for weighing. The average weight of the clothes should be evaluated and deducted from the measure. The weight is then recorded to the nearest 100 grams. Every morning the scale should be checked against a known 10 kg weight. If the measure does not match the weight, the springs must be changed or the scale discarded.

Height

Children who are more than two years old are measured while standing and younger children are measured while lying down. If exact age is unknown, as may be true with young unaccompanied minors, those children who are more than 85 centimeters (cm) are measured standing and those who are 85 cm or less are measured while lying down.

Either a measuring board can be made or children can be measured on a table that is marked for the head position. The assistant holds the sides of the child's head and positions the head against the headboard, which should be perpendicular to the table. The feet are placed against the footboard and the measurement is read. Children more than two years of age are encouraged to stand upright in the middle of the board. Ankles and knees are firmly pressed against a vertical measuring board while the measurer positions the head and the cursor. The child's head, shoulders, buttocks, knees and heels should be touching the board. The measurer reads the measurement to the nearest 0.1 cm. The assistant writes down the measurement and repeats it to the measurers to insure that it has been heard and recorded correctly.

Edema

Edema is an abnormal collection of fluid in the extracellular space of the body and is a sign of malnutrition. In order to measure edema, normal thumb pressure is applied to the foot or the leg for three seconds. If a shallow print or pit remains when the thumb is lifted, then the child has edema. The edema should be present on both of the child's feet or legs if it is caused by malnutrition.

Mid upper arm circumference

This measurement is used for children between one and five years of age. A mid upper arm circumference (MUAC) insertion tape is used. The thin end slips through the opening at the wider end and the measurement is read at the point indicated by the arrows. The MUAC is measured on the left arm at the mid-point between the elbow and shoulder. The measurement is read to the nearest 0.1 cm. MUAC may seem easier to measure than weight-for-height (WFH), but in fact more mistakes are made in measuring MUAC. Because of the variability among measurers for MUAC, we do not recommend using it if height and weight measurements can be done. If needed, the MUAC can be used to screen large numbers of children in search of those who may be malnourished. The standard MUAC measure denoting severe malnutrition is <12.5 cm.

Interpreting the measurements

In general one calculates the weight-for-age index, the weight-for-height index and the height-for-age index. These are compared to values for a reference population, usually to the reference values collected by the National Center for Health Statistics (NCHS) in the United States. In emergency situations where acute forms of malnutrition are the predominant pattern, the weight-for-height (WFH) index is the most appropriate to quantify levels of current acute malnutrition. The WFH index does not require age determination, which is often difficult to ascertain in a disaster situation.

The Centers for Disease Control (CDC), which is based in Atlanta, Georgia, has software that is user-friendly and excellent for calculating the anthropometric indices described, and may be used in a handheld computer. The results of these indices may be reported as percentages of the median, percentiles and/or Z scores. The Z scores express a child's weight or height as a multiple of the standard deviation (a measure of the spread of values around the mean) of the reference population, and are also known as "standard deviation scores." Z scores are more statistically correct than percentages of the reference group mean.

Estimating sample size

In general one chooses children between 6 and 59 months of age for a nutritional survey. Because they are growing rapidly, a diminished food supply will affect them first. Sample size is usually based on an expected prevalence of malnutrition between 5 and 20%. The formula for calculation of the sample size is the following:

$$n = t^2 \bullet (p \bullet q) / d^2$$

n = sample size

t = parameter related to the error risk, equals 1.96 or 2 for an error risk of 5%

p = the expected prevalence of malnutrition in the population, expressed as a fraction of 1.

q = 1 − p, the expected proportion of children without malnutrition, expressed as a fraction of 1.

d = the absolute precision, expressed as a fraction of 1.

In general, **t** is fixed to 1.96 and can be rounded up to 2. The expected prevalence is usually chosen to be closer to 50% than truly expected in order to get a sufficiently large sample size. Precision is arbitrary and can be modified.

For example, if expected malnutrition is 20% and desired precision is 3%, the sample size estimate is:

$$n = 1.96^2 \bullet (0.20 \bullet 0.80) / 0.03^2 = \mathbf{683}$$

Choosing a sampling frame

Sampling methods include random sampling, systematic sampling and cluster sampling. Systematic sampling can be used in well-organized refugee camps or in neighborhoods where houses are arranged in blocks and lines. One can then sample every nth household, where n is any whole number. Random sampling can be used if there is a list that includes every individual in the population, which is unlikely in the early states of a disaster. Names are drawn randomly from the list. A third method is two-stage cluster sampling. A number of clusters are randomly chosen, then a certain number of children are selected from each cluster and these children are surveyed. Within each cluster, children will have a tendency to be more similar to one another with respect to nutritional status. Therefore, the sample size should be twice as large for cluster sampling than it would be for random or systematic sampling.

Cluster sampling is most often used in the emergency phase of a disaster. The clusters or units may be villages, camp sections or specific geographical areas. The number of children to be selected in each cluster is determined by dividing the total sample size by the number of clusters. For example, the calculated sample size (from above) of 683 should be doubled to 1366 for cluster sampling. If the sampling frame uses 30 clusters, then 1366 divided by 30 equals approximately 45 children in each cluster.

When clusters are identified, the data collectors should go to the center of each cluster and choose a random direction by spinning a bottle. The surveyor walks in the direction indicated by the bottle, moving from the center to the border of the cluster, and counts the number of households encountered along the way. The first household to be visited is randomly selected from among these counted households by drawing a random number. The next nearest household available is selected until the required numbers of children in the cluster have been measured.

When survey information indicates that there is a serious health problem, it is essential that relief workers take the data to those in authority, make recommendations for reducing the health problem, and be advocates for children.

12. Sexual and Gender Based Violence

Sexual violence is a gross violation of basic human rights that is sometimes used as a weapon of war—forced impregnation leading to "ethnic cleansing," disruption of local communities by instilling terror, and as a means of torture and punishment. Types of violence may include rape, oral/anal coitus, forced marriage, infanticide, enforced sterilization, domestic violence, forced prostitution, female genital mutilation and honor killing. Such violence may occur after natural disasters as well as man made disasters.

Women and children, especially lone females and unaccompanied minors (both boys and girls) are most vulnerable to sexual violence. Militia members, bandits, guards and other refugees may attack them, and they may be captured to be used as sexual slaves. In the camp setting, security is a significant issue and attacks may occur while victims are in remote areas (i.e. gathering firewood, using latrines). During the reintegration phase they may be forced to have sex in exchange for supplies or ID cards, and cultural norms such as forced marriages and genital mutilation/circumcision may be reinstated.

Underreporting is a significant problem, since victims/survivors often are seen as bringing dishonor upon themselves or their family, and in many cultures the victim is viewed as the culprit and punished by imprisonment, torture or death while the attackers go unpunished. Frequently there is fear of reprisal by the attackers for reporting the event. In addition, there is an increase in the number of reports of peacekeeping forces and NGO workers who are involved with sexual violence toward refugees and internally displaced persons.

Physical effects include sexually transmitted infections (including HIV), mutilated genitalia, pregnancy, miscarriage, abortion and future infertility. Psychological effects include depression, anxiety, feelings of worthlessness, and denial. Children are particularly at high risk of developing long-term psychological and psychosocial problems as a result of sexual trauma. Children who are born of rape may be abandoned or killed.

The utmost regard should be taken to ensure the victim's physical safety and prevent any further suffering, and the victim's wishes should be respected in all instances. Strict confidentiality is crucial. Medical and psychosocial care should be provided using same-sex providers. A thorough examination of the victim should be done, including clothing and foreign matter. Antibiotics for Sexually Transmitted Infections should be given, and HIV/pregnancy risk should be addressed. Measures must be taken to ensure the safety of children and avoid repetition of the trauma. Prevention of sexual violence should begin by providing special accommodations for women and children and improving camp security in general as well as educating authorities and refugees. Host governments can enact strong policies against sexual violence and follow up with punishment of perpetrators.

Child sex trade

Over one million children per year worldwide are sold into sex trade through a variety of clandestine networks. In many parts of the world, up to 50% of prostitutes are children, even as young as 4 years of age. Children are at increased risk in situations of poverty, both natural and man-made disasters, domestic abuse, and as a result of being orphaned by AIDS. Many children are sold into brothels by parents or other family members. Other involved parties include community leaders, pimps and madams, and organized crime. The impact on children is lifelong in terms of both physical and psychological effects. Low self-esteem, shame and guilt, denial, nightmares, depression and a fear of men are often seen in rescued victims. There are a number of rescue organizations that provide medical treatment as well as education and job training, and several human rights organizations are working to enact legislation and promote awareness in various countries and cultures. It is essential that relief workers be aware of the possibility of both sexual violence and sex trading occurring in disasters, that they take preventive steps, and that they intervene when it occurs.

13. Epidemiology

The study of the distribution and determinants of disease frequency in human populations.

Epidemiology is a fundamental component of relief work. Although frequently thought of as the study of epidemics, field epidemiology involves:

- Gathering information on health problems.

- Identification of information sources.

- Gathering data, surveys.

- Presentation, statistical analysis and synthesis of data collected.

- Decision-making based on data results.

Epidemiological programs can be roughly divided into two categories: surveillance and ad hoc investigations. Epidemiological surveillance refers to the routine surveillance of health problems that serve as an early warning system for health care workers. Ad hoc investigations include the initial assessment/survey of a situation or epidemic.

Before initiating a survey, the goals and limitations of the investigation must be clearly delineated. Surveys are often considered essential in the early response to disasters. However, conducting a survey that is not followed by policy decisions is a waste of resources and raises false hopes among participants. The first consideration in implementing most surveys is to ascertain whether the person commissioning the study has the means to act on the results.

HEALTH INDICATORS

Due to constraints of time, money and people, it is unrealistic to collect all of the data that could possibly be used in following the evolution of an emergency. Instead, specific health indicators are used which are chosen for their relevance in describing a given situation or its evolution over time. In general, indicators are used that are directly related to health (morbidity, mortality, nutritional status) or to the environment (physical, economic, social, political or health care service environment).

A number of criteria are useful in selecting appropriate health indicators:

- Relevance to what the study is supposed to measure.

- Ability to be precisely defined.

- Ability to be analyzed in relationship to other parameters.

- Availability of a test to measure the effectiveness of the indicator.

SOURCES OF INFORMATION

After defining the type and number of indicators required, the epidemiologist must determine where the necessary data can be collected. The source of the data will be dependent on the type of information sought and details specific to the emergency situation. Possible sources include:

- The affected population being served.

- Administrative services.

- Community health services.

- Health care facilities.

- The humanitarian agencies.

DATA COLLECTION METHODS

Once epidemiologists have determined "what to collect" and "where to collect," they must decide how to collect the data. There are basically two choices: go out and look for it or wait for it to come to them. A number of factors influence the choice between these two, including:

- Time available for data collection.

- Physical access to information sources.

- Degree of reliability required.

- Degree of continuity required.

- Existence and status of a functional local health information system.

EFFECTIVENESS OF AN INDICATOR

When considering the effectiveness of an indicator, several characteristics should be considered:

- **Representativeness:** Does the indicator actually measure what you are looking for? For example, if concerned with measuring acute malnutrition, weight-for-height measurements would be an appropriate indicator. In contrast, weight-for-age measurements would reflect both acute and chronic malnutrition.

- **Standardization:** Is the same measuring method consistently used for a given indicator? Standardization allows one to compare data from different sources and different times.

- **Reliability:** Is the measure repeatable? Reliability is dependent upon the variation present in the instrument and in the item being measured. Reliability is affected by variation within the same measurer (intra-observer reliability) and by variation between different measurers (inter-observer reliability). In disaster situations, a number of unique factors may affect the reliability of an indicator, such as frequent changes in health care workers, rapid training of local personnel, and limited time to execute and plan the measuring activities.

- **Applicability:** Can the method for measuring the indicator be realistically used in the field during an emergency situation?

- **Acceptability:** Is the measure acceptable to the population being assessed and to the local authorities?

- **Validity:** How well does the indicator work? This is commonly reflected by the following expressions:

  - **SENSITIVITY = true positives ÷ (true positives + false negatives).**

  - **SPECIFICITY = true negatives ÷ (true negatives + false positives).**

  - **POSITIVE PREDICTIVE VALUE = true positives ÷ (true positives + false positives).**

Desirable qualities in a measure include representativeness, and reliability. Qualities that are particularly relevant in disaster situations include applicability and acceptability.

PRESENTATION OF DATA

The data collected must be converted into more usable forms, such as percentages, rates, tables and graphs. Most data should be expressed in the form of a rate, where the numerator represents the number of individuals affected (or the number of events that occurred) and the denominator represents the entire population of interest. Rates allow health care workers to follow trends, compare populations and conduct ongoing surveillance. The most commonly used rates in disasters are mortality rates, malnutrition rates and rates of incidence of the most common diseases. Humanitarian workers should become familiar with these.

Crude Mortality Rate (CMR), the most specific indicator of population health:

- Baseline   0.5 deaths/10,000/day

- Effective relief   < 1.0 deaths/10,000/day

- Serious   1.0 – 2.0 deaths/10,000/day
- Crisis   > 2.0 deaths/10,000/day

Under Five Mortality Rate (U5MR), for children under 5 years of age:

- Baseline   0.8 – 1.2 deaths/10,000/day
- Serious   > 4.0/10,000/day

Cause-Specific Mortality Rate, the proportion of deaths due to a specific disease:

- Used to measure effectiveness of interventions.

Case Fatality Rate, the proportion of individuals with a specific disease that die.

Age—and Sex—Specific Mortality Rates

- Calculated as secondary analyses.
- Defines populations at increased risk.

Acute malnutrition rate, calculated for children less than 5 years of age:

- Second most specific indicator of population health.
- Should include the prevalence of both acute protein-energy malnutrition and micronutrient deficiencies.

INCIDENCE AND PREVALENCE

Care must be taken to clearly identify rates as either incidence or prevalence, which are defined below:

- **Incidence:** the number of new cases that occur during a given period of time; provides information about the spread of disease, of particular concern in disasters.

- **Prevalence:** the number of cases present at a particular moment in time; useful for evaluating diseases of longer duration, such as tuberculosis.

STATISTICAL ANALYSIS AND TOOLS

Basic statistical analysis addresses three concepts: data distribution, sampling and statistical comparison. Data distribution refers to the variability and central tendencies of the study results obtained. Sampling refers to the manner in which a study population was chosen, such that study results are representative of the general population. Statistical comparison involves looking for differences in the study results obtained from different populations.

The initial analyses for data distribution focus on measures of central tendencies. These include the mean, median and/or mode. The most common measure used is the mean. The next step of analysis focuses on measures of variability, which include:

- **Mean deviation:** the summation of individual deviations ÷ by the number of observations.

- **Variance:** the summation of the squares of individual deviations ÷ by the number of observations.

- **Standard deviation:** the square root of the variance.

The standard deviation is used to create a distribution curve. Most health indicators will have a normal distribution, also called a Gaussian or bell-shaped curve, around a central mean. The area under the curve that is within ± 1, ± 2, ± 3, standard deviations represents 68%, 95% and 99% of the population respectively.

In order to obtain a sample that is representative of the population being studied, all of the people in the population being studied must have an equal chance of being included in the sample; this minimizes bias. There are many acceptable sampling methods, including:

- Simple random sampling.

- Stratified random sampling.

- Systematic sampling.

- Cluster sampling.

The size of the sample should be large enough to reduce sampling error to an acceptable level and small enough to be cost-effective. Calculation of sample size is dependent on the type of sampling employed. Sample size and sampling methods are discussed in more detail in the chapter on child health assessments. There are many resources available online to support simple size estimation.

Some common measures of comparison and statistical tests are listed here:

- **Relative risk:** the ratio between the rate of a variable expressed in two populations.

- **Odds ratio:** the ratio between the probability that a subject has been exposed to a risk factor and the probability that a control has been exposed to a risk factor.

- **Chi-squared test:** compares the number of individuals from two or more populations who do or do not possess the characteristics being studied.

- **Student's t-test:** compares two means from two samples taken from two populations.

- **Correlation coefficient:** describes the association between two variables as either evolving in the same direction (positive correlation) or evolving in the opposite direction (negative correlation).

- **Analysis of Variance (ANOVA):** compares the results of several sets of data by examining the variability between the sets of measures and the variability within each set.

Whenever a sample is used to describe a population, there is a certain risk of error. The results obtained will vary from the truth by some amount. The amount of error risk that is acceptable is pre-determined. In general, epidemiologists allow a 5% risk of accepting results that support a difference between two populations when in fact there is no difference (type I error). This risk is expressed as a probability, the p-value. The difference between two populations is significant when the probability of making a mistake is less than 5% ($p < 0.05$). Differences are highly significant when the probability of making a mistake is less than 1% ($p < 0.01$).

INTERPRETATION OF THE RESULTS

When data analysis is complete, epidemiologists must decide what their results mean. This begins with an assessment of whether the results are any good and whether they have been analyzed correctly. Factors to be considered in the critique of data collection methods include the relevancy of indicators, adequacy of sample size and accuracy of recording. Factors to be considered in the critique of statistical methods include confidence intervals and the appropriateness of the statistical test used. Epidemiologists must also consider the results in a broader context:

- Is the information pertinent to the current phase of the disaster?

- Do the data accurately describe the situation? Do the data represent all groups? Are the data reliable?

- In what context were the data collected? How might the data have been affected by local climate, the socio-cultural environment and population influx?

DECISION-MAKING

In disasters, the primary goal of epidemiological investigations is to facilitate fast decision making. Ultimately, the health care team can make one of the following choices based on the results of a survey:

- Do nothing.
- Carry out more specific investigations.
- Repeat the same study within a given period of time.
- Intervene immediately.

14.   Water and Sanitation

Effective water purification and sanitation programs are the most critical and fundamental elements of any relief operation in disasters. The relationships between the environment, water supply and disease are well accepted. Many diseases are associated with water shortages, contaminated water, poor sanitation and poor excreta disposal. In disasters, the establishment of effective water and sanitation programs decreases total mortality more than any other intervention. In a 1985 review of 67 studies from 26 countries, the impact of water supply and sanitation led to mean reductions in diarrhea morbidity of 22% and total mortality of 21%.

All health care workers should be able to understand and monitor the effects of water and sanitation programs in disasters. In particular, health care providers should be able to recognize the health problems related to ineffective water and sanitation programs and be familiar with the key elements of water and sanitation programs. They must be able to determine when a sanitation specialist is needed.

Water and sanitation programs should be established during the earliest phases of a crisis situation and must be maintained throughout the crisis. The promotion of sustainability should be incorporated into the initial plan. Community involvement in all phases of the plan is essential to ensure sustainability.

In the initial planning phase, community involvement will lead to the most culturally sensitive and acceptable programs. Water and sanitation programs that fail to address the cultural needs of a community will not be used. For example, the potable (drinkable) water supply must not only meet biological standards, but must be palatable and physically acceptable to those who drink it. In later phases, effective water and sanitation programs will require continual maintenance and monitoring. If the community has ownership of these programs, they are more likely to meet the maintenance needs of the programs.

The unique impact and needs of children must be considered when establishing water and sanitation programs. Children are the primary source of disease spread by the fecal-oral route. Not only do children have an increased incidence of these diseases, but they also have an increased burden of bacterial and parasitic loads. They are much less discrete with regards to urination and defecation. They will choose to relieve themselves in open, public spaces before traveling a significant distance or using a space that they may perceive as frightening. Also, children do not understand and are not concerned with careful hand washing. For these reasons, it is critical that latrines be readily available, child-friendly and near to an easily accessible water source for hand washing. Above all, children need consistent adult role models. Thus, effective hygiene education targeting all age groups is necessary.

WATER PURIFICATION PROGRAMS

The basic goals of effective water purification programs are to provide an adequate amount of safe water and to ensure fair distribution. Any water program is only as strong as the weakest of these links. The ideal amount of water supplied during a CHE is greatly determined by the phase of the disaster situation and the anticipated length of need. During the emergency phase of a disaster, the absolute minimum requirements for water must be met. Although greatly affected by exertion, physiologic minimums are 3 liters per person per day in temperate climates and 6–10 liters per person per day in hot climates.

As soon as possible, the water supply must be increased from these physiologic minimums. For example, a water supply of 20–25 liters is needed to maintain minimal hygiene. This requirement must be met if one hopes to impact health status. In order to maintain a field hospital, 35–40 liters per person per day must be provided. As a disaster situation evolves, or if a prolonged need is anticipated, other factors must be considered. Cultural variations in hygiene and cooking practices lead to very different water demands. Populations may have greatly increased water needs due to livestock. A cow drinks 30 liters of water per day! It is critical to use local experts to define immediate and long-term water needs.

The first step in providing safe water is to identify and protect available water sources. Currently used water sources must be identified and new water sources defined. All possible water sources should be considered, including rainwater, surface water, spring water and ground water. Once again, the contribution of local experts in this task is invaluable. It is critical that potential and existing water sources be protected from pollution. It is much more efficient to prevent pollution of a water source than to purify that same source.

Theoretically, the definition of safe water is determined by the anticipated use of that water. Potable water must be significantly more pure than water supplied for bathing and washing. It is well accepted that provision of an adequate amount of impure water has a greater impact on health than a small amount of pure water. Unfortunately, it is unrealistic to create two separate water supplies in most disaster situations. Thus, it is ideal to have all of the water supply be potable. In addition, there must be appropriate containers for transport of this water. The quality of the water supplied is irrelevant if the population being served uses contaminated buckets.

The definition of potable water is water that contains < **10 fecal coliform organisms per 100 ml**. Potable water must be both biologically and culturally acceptable. If the water is clean but cloudy, will people drink it? The three basic principles of water purification are settlement, filtration and disinfection. In general, a combination of these three approaches works best. Water purification through boiling is not practical for large populations, since boiling 1 liter of water requires ½ kilo of wood.

The main goal of settlement, also referred to as storage, is the removal of organic matter. This process may be facilitated by use of aluminum salts, which bind organic matter and speed up the sedimentation process. Less disinfection is required when organic matter is removed at this stage of the purification process. Also, certain pathogens may be eliminated merely by the passage of time. For example, cercariae that transmit schistosomiasis die within 48 hours.

Although there are a variety of filtration methods, sand filtration is the most common approach. Slow sand filtration (0.2 m/hr) is based on the principle of natural filtration through the soil. Water is purified as it passes through alternating layers of sand, gravel and charcoal.

Disinfection refers to the addition of chemicals to water in order to eliminate organic matter. Careful control over this process is essential. By far, the most commonly used disinfectant is chlorine. When using chlorination, several basic principles should be remembered. Five milliliters of 1% chlorine will treat 20 liters of water. Five milliliters is about one teaspoon, although some teaspoons are smaller than this. There are many preparations of chlorine; this dosage refers to the amount of free chlorine added. Thus, the effective dose of free chlorine is 0.5 mg/liter, acting over a period of half an hour. Over-chlorination will lead to toxicity.

The most difficult element to create in a water purification program is fair distribution. Without community leaders advocating for equitable water use, success is unattainable. In unsuccessful situations, it is the most vulnerable members of the population who are denied access to water. In some situations, it may be necessary to establish a community-managed guard system over the water supply. Consideration must be given to areas requiring disproportionate amounts of water, such as hospitals, health centers and fire fighting facilities. There should always be a reserve of water in case an interruption occurs in the current water supply.

SANITATION

The single most effective control measure of infectious disease spread is proper sanitation. In general, there are two modes of transmission of infectious disease: direct contact and environmental contact. Transmission through direct contact is most effectively decreased through the supply of adequate amounts of water and the promotion of good hygiene. For example, surfaces such as dishes, stethoscopes, ties, toys and pens often contain disease-causing pathogens. Transmission through the environment can occur via water, food, soil, insects and air. All of these elements must be considered when developing sanitation programs.

The rate of infectious disease transmission by the fecal route is directly affected by the quantity and quality of excreta produced. Although it is impossible to control the quantity of excreta produced, it is possible to affect the quality of the excreta. Based on the phase of the emergency, it may be appropriate to chemically treat the infected individuals and thereby decrease the spread and prevalence of disease. In certain situations, it may be appropriate to implement prophylactic treatment to decrease the carrier rate. Infection and medication must be considered individually in every situation. For instance, the treatment of severe intestinal helminthic infections can lead to the development of bowel obstruction and perforation. This is a particular risk for children. Thus, in a transient, mobile population with lack of access to adequate medical facilities, it would be inappropriate to treat children for intestinal helminthic infections without first examining them.

When designing sanitation programs, the key considerations are similar to those relevant to developing water programs: cultural sensitivity, community involvement and health education.

There are many factors associated with the cultural acceptance of sanitary facilities, regardless of type. It has been estimated that only 20% of rural populations in developing countries had access to sanitary facilities. With this in mind, it is not surprising that people will frequently find it unclean to defecate in an area that someone else has already used. People tend to search for areas that provide some level of privacy. Keeping latrines open to sunlight makes them more appealing for human use, but also increases fly infestation. Children are sometimes afraid of using latrines because they believe that they will fall in the open receptacle. Some simple considerations may alleviate a significant portion of these issues: the designation of male and female areas, using some form of barrier and creating stable surfaces around latrines.

Community involvement is even more important in sanitation programs than in water programs. In general, sanitation programs require less technology than water purification. Thus, the community can be involved at all levels of the program, including design, construction and maintenance. In reality, there is a much greater need for prolonged, intensive maintenance in sanitation programs than in water programs. Since the maintenance associated with sanitation programs is not the most pleasant duty, the community will be much more responsive to meet this need if they have ownership in the project.

The success of sanitation programs hinges upon effective educational programs. In many situations, sanitation programs do not parallel societal norms. People frequently view use of sanitation facilities as bothersome, unclean and unnecessary. If a population is expected to make significant behavioral changes, they must have seen a convincing presentation of the necessity. Without a strong, fundamental educational component, sanitation programs will fail. Educational programs can be tailored to bridge the gap of cultural acceptability. For example, topics may be effectively presented through school children, puppets, pantomime or parades.

There are several approaches to developing sanitation programs. The choice of which technique to employ should be based on the phase of the emergency, anticipated need, environment and cultural acceptability. Immediate precautions should focus on separation and containment. Separation refers to keeping excreta separate from the water and food supply. People frequently view water sources, such as riverbanks, streams and ponds, as ideal places to defecate. Even if not currently needed, these water sources will often become needed with increasing population demands on the water supply. Fields with crops are also viewed as an ideally private area to relieve oneself. This too increases the rate of disease transmission.

Instead of identifying areas that are inappropriate for use, it is much easier to specify appropriate areas for defecation and urination. This is the basis of containment. The simplest application of this theory is creating defecation fields. These are designated areas for excreta, which are located at significant distance from areas of high traffic, food preparation and water supply. If possible, these areas should have some barrier for privacy. Also, it is critical that defecation fields are located downhill from living areas in order to avoid contamination of the water table.

A full description of intermediate and long-term measures for sanitation is beyond the scope of this manual. Intermediate measures consist of various latrine forms, including family, communal and trench latrines. Of these options, family latrines are the best choice for several reasons. Since used by a small group of individuals, they minimize the rate of infectious disease spread. Also, this form of latrine tends to promote ownership and results in the best maintenance. When a prolonged need for sanitation programs is anticipated, pit latrines offer the ideal long-term solution. This type of latrine is superior in terms of excreta removal and community acceptance, but is more costly and requires a higher level of technical skill.

The Sphere Handbook: Humanitarian Charter and Minimum Standards in Humanitarian Response is available in English as well as in many other language versions. It contains minimum standards for water quantity and quality, excreta disposal, vector control, solid waste management and drainage. www.sphereproject.org

15.   Warmth, Clothing, Housing

Morbidity and mortality are increased among children who lack adequate warmth, clothing and housing in disasters. Unaccompanied children are especially vulnerable to these problems. Without family advocates, they are likely to be displaced from the best available shelters, to have clothing and blankets stolen, and to lack access to stoves or fires. The risk is even higher for those malnourished children who lack subcutaneous fat stores.

In the Goma refugee situation of 1994, the lack of clothing and blankets combined with rainy, cool weather resulted in unaccompanied infants and toddlers dying from low core body temperatures. During the movement of refugees back to Rwanda in December 1996, there were 400,000 children (90% of children) who lacked footwear, while 75% of adult males and 60% of adult females had shoes. As a result of walking long distances barefoot, the children suffered tissue breakdown on the soles of their feet with rapid invasion by "jiggers" and subsequent deep infections, including osteomyelitis.

Fear and anxiety can reduce the core body temperature of children. A study sponsored by the National Institutes of Health (NIH) showed that core temperatures of newly hospitalized children dropped two degrees during the first 48 hours of hospitalization. The temperature drop was attributed to stressors such as strangers, laboratory procedures and a strange environment. Displaced children also experience fear and anxiety, which may place them at risk for lower core body temperatures.

During movements of displaced people there may be no alternative but to sleep out in the open. The best way to provide warmth for children is for them to sleep next to their parents or other children in an area that is out of the wind. Priority should be given to using available clothing and blankets for the smallest and most malnourished of young children. Hay, grass and straw, if available, can be used to provide warmth while sleeping. Plastic sheets can be cut up into makeshift clothing or blankets that will hold body heat. Studies of "kangaroo" holding of infants by their mothers (i.e. skin to skin against the chest and abdomen) have found that this is an effective way to warm and nurture even premature infants.

Shoes, of the zōri or flip-flop variety, can be made out of old rubber tires or constructed from wood, if these materials are available. While it is generally desirable to bathe children, this is not recommended in cold situations where there is lack of heat, clothing and shelter.

Bathing results in a decrease of core temperature that may be harmful if the child cannot be re-warmed immediately. If bathing of children is done outside, this should occur at the warmest time of the day.

If tents or other temporary type shelters are available, they should be set up in such a way that snow or rain moves away from the structure. Desert tents can be modified for use in a rainy situation. Shelters made of plastic sheeting and poles can provide useful, temporary housing. Nursing mothers, young children and especially unaccompanied minors, should receive priority in assignment of whatever shelters are available.

16. Nutrition

In 2008 the WHO estimated that 5 million children die of malnutrition every year, and that over half of all child deaths are associated with malnutrition. Children less than 5 years of age are among the most acutely affected by undernutrition. The evolution of malnutrition is complex and strongly linked to many social and economic factors that are frequently triggered by natural disasters. A famine is defined as occurring when food consumption is reduced to the point of leading to acute malnutrition and increasing mortality. A nutrition emergency is defined as when there is the risk of or an actual rise in mortality from malnutrition. In the past few decades armed conflict instead of natural disasters has increasingly become the main cause of nutrition emergencies. Children affected by disasters are particularly vulnerable to all forms of malnutrition, including both protein energy malnutrition (PEM) and micro-nutrient deficiencies.

MALNUTRITION

Malnutrition in children is manifested by growth failure and undernutrition. Undernutrition may be due to stunting (low height-for-age) and/or wasting (low weight-for-height). Stunting is a feature of chronic malnutrition, and while many wasted children also suffer from stunting, the focus in emergencies is on acute malnutrition (wasting) because of its stronger link with immediate mortality. Acute malnutrition is divided into the categories of severe acute malnutrition (SAM) and moderate acute malnutrition (MAM). MAM is defined as a weight-for-height between 2 and 3 standard deviations below the reference population median without edema. SAM is defined as a weight-for-height of more than 3 standard deviations below the reference population median, by visible severe wasting, and/or by the presence of edema.

Protein energy malnutrition (PEM) can refer to either acute or chronic undernutrition and includes both kwashiorkor and marasmus. The occurrence of PEM in populations affected by disasters is well recognized. Areas of humanitarian emergencies also often have high levels of chronic malnutrition and cases of higher prevalence of HIV/AIDS, which predispose to more severe nutrition emergencies. Marasmus is defined as a weight-for-height of less than three standard deviations of the reference population. Kwashiorkor is defined by the presence of bilateral edema of both feet, and children may not initially appear underweight because of their edema.

The word kwashiorkor originates from an African language, meaning "disease of the deposed or separated child." Kwashiorkor often occurs during the toddler period when a child has been deposed from the mother's breast by a new sibling. Children with kwashiorkor have a height and a weight that are lower than expected for their age. They appear lethargic and miserable and tend to move very little. Their unsmiling faces have "chipmunk" or swollen cheeks. Muscles, especially of the upper arms and buttocks, are wasted, weak and atrophic. Skin appears dry and roughened, and there are areas that appeared to be burned. Edema is noticeable on lower extremities. Hair is dry, sparse and sometimes appears blonde or red in usually dark-haired children. Full-blown kwashiorkor is easy to diagnose; the clinician should note earlier signs of malnutrition such as lightening of hair roots, decreased elasticity of external ears and apathy.

Children with marasmus generally appear emaciated or wizened. Muscle wasting is striking, and the child's skeleton is often visible. They demonstrate hair and skin changes less frequently than do children with kwashiorkor. They are more likely to act hungry, although they can appear apathetic as well. Clinically, children may present with symptoms from both kwashiorkor and marasmus.

Whenever PEM has been identified, concurrent micronutrient deficiencies are likely. A child with micronutrient deficiencies may actually have a normal weight-for-age, but display edema, hair and skin changes. Micronutrient deficiencies also play a key role in nutrition-related morbidity and mortality. Micronutrient deficiencies, manifested by diseases such as scurvy or iron deficiency anemia, have been consistently reported in refugee populations.

BREASTFEEDING

In nutrition emergencies, breastfeeding is a life-saving measure. Outbreaks of diseases associated with poor sanitation and compromised access to clean water make breastfeeding the most practical method of feeding infants and young children. Exclusive breastfeeding is recommended for the first 6 months of life and complementary foods can be introduced thereafter. This recommendation also includes HIV-infected or status unknown mothers, although if replacement feeding is acceptable, feasible, affordable, sustainable, and safe (AFASS) then it is preferred in order to reduce HIV transmission. However, in crisis settings it is unlikely that all of these requirements will be met, and studies have demonstrated increased mortality in infants who are replacement fed in settings of inadequate access to clean water, societal prejudices, etc. In crisis settings there will be some infants who have lost mothers or who have mothers without milk due to stress. If surrogate mothers with breast milk cannot be found, then these infants must be given formula feeds. These should be given with a cup and spoon, not with a feeding bottle.

The most basic step in preventing PEM and micronutrient deficiencies is to promote breastfeeding throughout the first two years of life. The following is a brief highlight of selected benefits from breast milk:

- Protects and promotes infant health by augmenting the infant's immature immune system from birth into the second year of life.

- Contains antibodies directed against many infectious agents, including shigella, salmonella, cholera, rotavirus, RSV, poliovirus, influenza, giardia and candida.

- The protein composition correlates with the ability of the infant's digestive tract to absorb various proteins. As the child's digestive tract develops, the composition of breast milk changes to parallel the digestive abilities of the child.

- Provides for 100% of energy needs up until 6 months of age. At 12 months of age, breast milk may provide for up to 35% of the infant's total energy intake.

- Breastfeeding has many psychological benefits, including the promotion of maternal-infant bonding and the empowerment of women over their situation.

- Breastfed children may graduate immediately from the breast to a cup. This avoids the use of bottles, which can transmit infectious diseases.

- All of the necessary nutrients and water are provided by breast milk for the first 6 months of an infant's life with the exception of:

  - Vitamin K – ideally given as an injection after birth.

  - Vitamin D – only necessary if the child is exposed to less than 30 minutes per week of sunlight.

  - Fluoride – required after 6 months of age, in areas where the water is not fluoridated.

  - Vitamin B12 – if mothers are strict vegetarians.

In light of the advantages afforded by breast milk, breastfeeding should be the option of choice in most situations. In less industrialized countries and in all disasters, the risk of infectious disease secondary to bottle-feeding outweighs the risk associated with breastfeeding, even when using wet nurses.

There are many factors that affect the success of breastfeeding, including maternal stress, hydration, nutritional status and the frequency of suckling. Thus, lactating and pregnant women should be recognized as vulnerable populations. Pregnant and lactating women need increased rations of food and water and should receive iron/folic acid supplements. In stable populations, these women must be carefully evaluated for enrollment in supplemental feeding programs. In transient populations, pregnant and lactating women should be transported along with other vulnerable populations when at all possible and provided appropriate nutrition.

PREVENTION AND TREATMENT OF MALNUTRITION

Prevention and treatment of acute malnutrition in emergencies is usually conducted through general food distribution (GFD) programs, which target all households with a food ration, and selective feeding programs that target specific groups. Selective feeding programs are furthermore divided into Supplementary Feeding Programs (SFPs) to manage MAM and inpatient or outpatient/community-based Therapeutic Feeding Programs (TFPs) to manage SAM. When it is possible, SFPs should be linked with TFPs and other existing health infrastructure in addition to livelihood programs such as cash or voucher assistance.

It is important to identify potential nutrition emergencies early on in order to take timely action as needed. Instructions for nutritional surveys are given in the chapter on child health assessments. During the initial assessment period, rapid nutrition surveys must be completed. After they are completed, more thorough assessments can be completed in conjunction with a supplemental feeding program. Anthropometric indicators of acute and severe malnutrition are late indicators, and should not be used to predict a nutrition emergency. Early warning indicators instead could include reduced rainfall, food shortages, loss of livestock, increase in food prices, epidemics, etc.

Table 1 adopted from Johns Hopkins/IFRC provides recommended actions with respect to the level of malnutrition.

Table 1: Nutrition Surveillance Benchmarks

Nutrition Situation	Recommended Actions
Acute malnutrition rate >15% or 10–14% with aggravating factors *	Emergency food aid; general food ration Blanket supplementary feeding Therapeutic feeding of severely malnourished individuals
Acute malnutrition rate 10–14% or 5–9% with aggravating factors*	No general rations Targeted supplementary feeding Therapeutic feeding of severely malnourished
Acute malnutrition rate <10% with no aggravating factors	No emergency food and nutrition intervention

- Aggravating factors include: household food insecurity, high prevalence HIV/AIDS, crude mortality rate > 1/10,000/day, under-five crude mortality > 2/10,000/day, epidemic of measles or pertussis, high prevalence of respiratory or diarrheal diseases, high prevalence of pre-existing malnutrition (e.g. stunting).

- Blanket supplementary feeding provides food supplement to all members of a specified at risk group, regardless of whether they have MAM.

- Targeted supplementary feeding provides support to individuals with MAM. They generally target children under five, malnourished pregnant and breastfeeding mothers, and other nutritionally at-risk individuals.

There have been several studies in the past decade which have demonstrated that MAM and SAM, without medical complications can be treated at home, using Ready to Use Therapeutic Foods (RUTF). In the first trials of RUTF peanuts were the basis for the nutrient dense, palatable food containing micronutrients. RUTF have a similar nutrient composition to F100 with the exception of water and iron. RUTF do not contain water in order to reduce bacterial growth. They can be used at home without refrigeration. WHO has developed international standards to be used in the manufacturing of RUTF; these include nutrition composition and safety guidelines. WHO has also developed protocols for facility based management of SAM, using treatments which include RUTF. This has improved the quality of hospital care.

When children are treated with this approach, they require regular monitoring at a health facility. They should be provided RUTF until adequate weight has been gained. In some communities the RUTF may be developed, using locally available nutrient dense foods with added micronutrients.

The management of the child with severe malnutrition is divided into four phases:

1. Stabilization phase: Children are treated for acute illnesses, The stabilization phase requires 24-hour care and typically lasts 1–7 days. Medical care focuses on rehydration, initiation of nutritional treatment and medical treatment. The main causes of death in severe PEM are addressed during the first phase of supplemental feeding programs. These include dehydration, infection, hypothermia, hypoglycemia, cardiac failure and severe anemia. Therapeutic feeding is begun with F75.

Fluids must be given cautiously. Use oral rehydration in frequent, small amounts whenever possible. Monitor the patient's weight, edema, temperature, urine frequency, pulse and respiratory rate. Development of eyelid edema or pulmonary crackles may indicate that the child is overhydrated. Children with kwashiorkor are usually over-hydrated and shouldn't be treated for dehydration unless there is a clear history of watery diarrhea. Hypothermia and hypoglycemia are also particularly important complications in phase one. Many malnourished children are irritable and do not want to eat. If necessary, they must be fed via nasogastric tubes.

Nearly all children suffering from SAM are suffering from infection. The most common infections encountered are respiratory tract infections, urinary tract infections, measles, gastrointestinal infections, malaria, skin infections and septicemia (bacterial infections of the blood). Children with PEM are often given multiple drugs for concurrent infections. There is evidence of impaired drug metabolism in malnourished children and some antibiotics impair intestinal absorption of nutrients. For example, aminoglycoside antibiotics impair absorption of amino acids; sulfa drugs delay gastric emptying. Before giving medications, the clinician should ask, "How may these drugs inhibit the nutritional rehabilitation of this child?"

2. Transition phase: This begins when the child has an appetite and edema is reduced. Therapeutic feeding moves from F75 to F100 and/or RUTF. Antibiotics are continued.

3. Rehabilitation phase: This may take place in either the inpatient or outpatient settings. The child's caregiver is taught how to continue care at home. Physical and emotional stimulation are provided the child and therapeutic feeding continues.

4. Follow up phase: After discharge children are examined regularly in home or clinic to document continued growth. Continued support is provided to caretakers, including teaching about appropriate foods, food preparation, encouragement of breast feeding, and appropriate play activities. Siblings should also be assessed for their nutritional status.

During Stabilization Phase

Most persons experienced in treating PEM are impressed with the efficacy of milk in the initial weeks of treatment. In SAM, renal dysfunction makes standard rehydration solutions dangerous due to potential hypernatremia and heart failure. Other protein preparations are cheaper but have qualitative deficiencies. If possible, milk-based treatment should be used for the first month of rehabilitation. F75 and F100 are commonly used therapeutic milks that can be obtained through UNICEF. One packet of F75 or F100 is dissolved in 2 L of water. A suggested therapeutic feeding protocol as adopted from the Johns Hopkins/IFRC for the severely malnourished child is as follows:

Therapeutic Feeding Protocol

PHASE ONE:	Step 1: Initiation of Re-feeding • -Eight feeds of F75 per day. Breastfed children should be breastfed before they are fed F75. • -The total amount of F75 (75 kcal/100 mL) to feed is 100 kcal/kg of body weight/day. • -Nasogastric tubes should be used for anorexic children who do not feed sufficiently by mouth • -If no F75 is available, F100 diluted in 2.7 L instead of 2 L can be used. Step 2: Administration of Routine Medicines • -Treatment of vitamin A deficiency if in Vitamin A deficient area • -Treatment of malaria if in an endemic area • -Antibiotics: first line is amoxicillin • -Folate 5 mg on the first day • -Oral iron supplements to treat severe anemia should NOT be given in Phase 1
TRANSITION PHASE:	The criteria to move from phase one to the transition phase are the return of appetite and the loss of edema in cases of kwashiorkor. The only change in treatment is to give F100 instead of F75. The number of feeds, timing, and amounts remain the same as in phase one. Patients should remain in transition phase for about 2 days.

REHAB AND FOLLOW UP	The goal is to allow the child to eat according to appetite and regain weight rapidly in a home or daycare setting.
	• Breastfed children should receive breast milk before F100
	• Six feeds should be given per day.
	• The total amount to feed is 150–220 kcal/kg of body weight/day
	• Children should be encouraged to eat but not force-fed
	• Iron supplementation, de-worming medicine, and measles vaccination should be given
	• Porridge or RUTF can be fed after F100

Discharge from an inpatient program is appropriate when at least 80% of median weight-for-height international standards are met and no edema is present. Discharge should be 85% weight-for-height if no supplementary feeding program is available.

REFEEDING AND LONGTERM EFFECTS

Each treatment unit must develop a protocol for refeeding that is consistent with the available foods and the available nursing care. Malnourished children recover much better with oral feedings; essential regeneration and hypertrophy of the intestinal mucosa do not occur with parenteral feeding.

It is important that all supplemental feeding programs be continually monitored for effectiveness. Parameters by which the effectiveness of feeding programs can be measured include attendance rates, mean length of stay, recovery rates, deaths, defaulters and relapse rates. Also, it is important to maintain continued nutritional surveillance of the general population. Using this data, it is possible to calculate the coverage rate of a feeding center. The coverage rate refers to that proportion of children, out of all of those suffering from severe malnutrition, who are participating in the supplemental feeding program.

The long-term consequences of severe malnutrition are devastating to both the individual and the community. During the first half of gestation and the first three years of life, brain development occurs which is crucial to focusing attention and inhibition. These are skills that are integral to planning, problem solving and sound critical judgment. Evidence from many studies suggests a causal relationship between undernutrition and behavioral development. In the seminal work completed by Dr. Janina Galler, 65% of children who had one episode of severe malnutrition during the first year of life had subsequent problems in learning and attention by the age of 9 to 10 years. Dr. Galler has now followed this cohort until past 40 years and has documented continued cognitive and coping problems. These long-term outcomes of early malnutrition may affect millions of adolescent and adult survivors of malnutrition. Rapid recognition and treatment of malnutrition in disasters is important to prevent these long-term effects.

References

The Johns Hopkins and International Federation of Red Cross and Red Crescent Societies Public Health Guide for Emergencies. 2nd Edition. 2008.

Wendy S. Garrett. Kwashiorkor and the Gut Microbiota. N Engl J Med 2013; 368:1746–1747.

The Harmonised Training Package (HTP): Resource Material for Training on Nutrition in Emergencies, Version 2 (2011). NutritionWorks, Emergency Nutrition Network, Global Nutrition Cluster.

WHO. Essential Nutrition Actions: improving maternal, newborn, infant and child health and nutrition, 2013.

Save The Children. Food for thought: tackling child malnutrition to unlock potential and boost prosperity. 2013

Galler JR, Ramsey FA. A follow-up study of the influence of early malnutrition on development: behavior at home and at school. J Amer Acad Child Adoles Psychiatry 28:254–261, 1989.

Waber DP, Eaglesfield D, Fitzmaurice GM, Bryce C, Harrison RH, and Galler JR. Cognitive impairment as a mediator in the developmental pathway from infant malnutrition and adolescent depressive symptoms in Barbadian youths. J. Devel Behav Pediatrics 12:225–232, 2011.

17.   Development and Mental Health

Man-made disasters are associated with higher levels of developmental and psychological trauma than are natural disasters. War may cause a child to experience the death of a loved one, loss of home and possessions, and relocation from familiar surroundings. This can also occur after natural disasters; however children are more likely to encounter loving adults and assistance immediately after a natural disaster. War results in many children witnessing brutal acts of violence to themselves or to family members. In both man-made and natural disasters, the distress for a child is compounded by the fact that his/her security system, the parents, are also experiencing loss, stress, fear and grief. These feelings are transmitted to the child who then feels more vulnerable.

DEVELOPMENTAL RESPONSES TO TRAUMA

Note that these typical responses to disasters may vary according to the culture and prior living situations.

Toddlers

- Reaction is often like that of parents.
- Regression in behaviors
- (e.g. may forget toilet training).
- Decreased appetite.
- Nightmares.
- Muteness.
- Clinging.
- Irritability.
- Exaggerated startle responses.

School-Age Children

- Marked reactions of fear and anxiety.
- Increased hostility with siblings.
- Somatic complaints
- (e.g. stomach aches).
- Sleep disorders.
- School problems.
- Decreased interest in peers, hobbies, school.
- Social withdrawal.
- Apathy.
- Reenactment via play.
- Post-traumatic stress disorder.

Preadolescents

- Increased hostility with siblings.
- Somatic complaints.
- Eating disorders.
- Sleep disorders.
- Decreased interest in peers, hobbies, and school.
- Rebellion.
- Refusal to do chores or to help.
- Interpersonal difficulties.
- Post-traumatic stress disorder.

Adolescents

- Decreased interest in social activities.
- Decreased interest in peers, hobbies, school.
- Anhedonia.
- Decline in responsible behaviors.

- Rebellion, behavior problems.
- Somatic complaints.
- Sleep disorders.
- Eating disorders.
- Change in physical activity (either increase or decrease).
- Confusion.
- Lack of concentration.
- Risk-taking behaviors.
- Post-traumatic stress disorder.

POST-TRAUMATIC STRESS DISORDER

The diagnosis of post-traumatic stress disorder (PTSD) is made when the child or adolescent has symptoms in each of the following three areas for more than one month:

Re-experiencing the event through play, nightmares or flashbacks; distress with events that resemble or symbolize the trauma.

Routine avoidance of reminders of the event.

Increased arousal or hypervigilance.

WEATHER PHOBIA

Weather phobia is a frequent sequela in children who have experienced natural disasters. Children with weather phobia become anxious when they perceive that there is a likelihood of a storm. They over react to benign clouds in the sky, running inside and crying. Some refuse to attend school or leave home at all because of these fears.

MENTAL HEALTH PROBLEMS

In disaster situations it is important to monitor children and adolescents for symptoms of psychological trauma and to intervene when they occur. Such monitoring can be done via teachers, indigenous healers, community health workers, food servers, and others. It is important to inform these people about the special mental health risks to children and how to help them.

One approach is to talk with parents and caretakers about their children. Do they note significant changes in a child's behavior? Are children confused and upset? If the children are toddlers, do they cry constantly or are they mute? Do they manifest head banging and rocking or other self-stimulatory behaviors? Are they unresponsive to physical contact? Do they show developmental regression? Another approach is to observe children at play. Does the play seem normal? Are children acting out recent events of the disaster? Are children speaking? What types of drawings are they making? Individuals who work in disasters should also pay close attention to signs of severe depression in mothers including lethargy or hyperactivity, inability to care for children, problems sleeping, frequent weeping and loss of appetite. Maternal depression is associated with concomitant symptoms in their children.

THE RESILIENCE PROJECT

Dr. Edith Grotberg defines resilience as a "universal capacity which allows a person, group or community to prevent, minimize or overcome the damaging effects of adversity." The purpose of the international resilience project is to promote resilience in children around the world. There are interactions between culture and resilience factors. Some cultures are more concerned with discipline and reconciliation; others are more concerned with punishment and guilt. Some cultures expect children to be dependent on others for help in adversity; others expect children to be self-reliant at an earlier age. Parents in some countries maintain close relationships with their children well into adolescence and other cultures do not. Regardless of these differences there are three sources of resilience ideas for children in most stable cultures: "I HAVE, I AM, I CAN."

I HAVE:

- People around me I trust and who love me, no matter what.
- People who set limits for me so I know when to stop before there is danger or trouble.

- People who show me how to do things right.
- People who want me to learn to do things on my own.
- People who help me when I am sick, in danger, or need to learn.

In disaster situations children often lose the adult support described under "I HAVE." This leads to their being overwhelmed by the adversities of disasters.

I AM:

- A person people can like and love.
- Glad to do nice things for others and show my concern.
- Respectful of myself and others
- Willing to be responsible for what I do.
- Sure things will be all right.

In disaster situations children may lack role models for the ideal personal qualities listed. They are at risk for never having the opportunity to develop such qualities and for becoming antisocial adults.

I CAN:

- Talk to others about things that frighten or bother me.
- Find ways to solve problems I face.
- Control myself when I feel like doing something not right or dangerous.
- Figure out when it is a good time to talk to someone or to take action.
- Find someone to help me when I need it.

In disasters children may not find respected adults who can help them to do the things listed or to feel secure. They then can have difficulties coping as they grow older because they have not had opportunities to practice problem solving with adult assistance, to develop self-control, or to talk with trusted people about things that bother them.

Even in the disaster setting, resilience can be promoted in children. Any person or staff providing services (I HAVE) can attempt to connect each child to a trusting, loving older person. Any person working with children can praise their accomplishments, show love and empathy, and encourage their hope and confidence (I AM). And any person, especially in educational settings, can help children master skills (I CAN).

MENTAL HEALTH INTERVENTIONS

Factors that improve the mental health of refugee or internally displaced children include:

- A return to the security that a stable family offers.

- Living in a stable environment that does not change from day to day.

- Provision of material needs such as food, water, medical care, and clothing.

- Organized education programs.

- Some understanding of what has happened and why, especially for the older children.

- The opportunity to complete all normal stages of child development.

- Opportunities and time to play.

- A belief in the future and the opportunity to influence what happens to them.

- Time and opportunity to recover after their experiences and to grieve over deaths of those who were close to them.

The World Health Organization (WHO) has published an excellent manual on mental health of refugees (see the chapter on resources). It provides guidance about how non-mental health professionals can learn to help refugees who are suffering mentally. It includes guidelines for teaching relaxation exercises, simple massage and breathing exercises, as well as ways to recognize serious psychological or psychiatric disorders. It discusses how to involve traditional healers in mental health treatment, how to help victims of rape or torture and how to help the children. The WHO manual emphasizes that mental health records require careful thought. They should reflect the child's culture and should include no information that could threaten or harm the child or the child's family. The United Nations High Commissioner for Refugees (UNHCR) suggests that diagnostic labels should not be given to adults or to children. Records should just describe the behavior. For example, "Child C is often seen crying during the day and is refusing food," or "Child A cannot sit still in school and does not do any work in school."

TENDER LOVING CARE

Children involved in disaster are at high risk for both physical and psychological sequelae. The consequences may affect their personalities, behaviors, learning abilities and adult work over a lifetime. Some of the negative psychological outcomes can be prevented or mitigated by rapid, early interventions. Most importantly, children need tender, loving care (TLC). The components of TLC involve the whole family and community:

Provide encouragement and support to parents. This can include arranging for home visitors, developing groups for mothers and young children to discuss the new problems of raising children in a disaster setting, and teaching ways to stimulate children in difficult disaster environments. The latter includes how to make toys from local materials. Mothers can benefit from day care programs that provide a few hours of care and stimulation for their preschool children. In day care, children can join in group play activities, including singing, dancing and games that use simple props. We have used empty plastic bottles to make puppets, or grass and sticks to make dolls, etc. In cultures that have traditions of handiwork such as making baskets, musical instruments or sewing, it is helpful to get materials for these activities and offer them to both adults and children.

Support breastfeeding mothers with food, liquid and emotional support so that they, in turn, are able to provide sustenance to their infants. By reducing the stress on lactating mothers, the breast milk supply will improve.

Find reliable 24-hour caretakers for unaccompanied minors, especially for those under school age. The caretakers should be female and can include adolescent refugee girls, volunteers from NGOs, older siblings in families who have lost their parents and elderly women. The caretakers, ideally, should be of the same ethnic group and speak the same language. However, if this is not possible, then a loving person of another ethnic group and speaking different language, is preferable to no caretaker. Providing such caretakers is urgent, especially for children under two years. Infants and toddlers do not survive in disasters if they lack 24-hour loving, attentive caretakers. Encouragement, recognition and support must be provided to the caretakers as well. Supervising health workers should observe caretakers to be certain that they are not abusing the children under their care.

Mental health support includes feeding. Young children must be fed frequently. Ideally, toddlers should be fed 4–5 times a day. The nurturing associated with feedings is especially important to the youngest children in disasters.

TLC includes bathing children, playing with them, talking with them, carrying those who cannot walk, helping them with toileting in a sanitary manner and maintaining routines as much as possible.

Organized efforts to identify local leaders, religious leaders and healers are important. Such individuals, who are respected and who know the language and culture can be helpful in addressing and reducing the emotional problems of children.

Many children are helped by the opportunity to talk about what they have witnessed, to act out what they have experienced or to make drawings. Caretakers should not interfere with a child's repetitive post-traumatic talk and play, unless it is dangerous.

Adolescents involved in disasters can benefit most from being involved in school and community activities. A sense of responsibility and purpose leads to an improved sense of personal competence, mastery and hope.

Return to Happiness Program

This program was developed by UNICEF in 1992 to help children who experienced humanitarian emergencies in Mozambique. It has since been adapted and used in Colombia, Nicaragua, and many other countries. The program includes a step by step process of helping children to cope with their lives after disasters. It involves training of community assistants and collaboration with local schools. The program includes provision of "psychosocial backpacks" to children which, depending on the local culture, contain appropriate toys, musical instruments, games and drawing materials.

(See List of Resources)

Child to Child Program

This program was created in the 70s by Professor David Morley to teach older children how to care for younger siblings. In recent years it has been modified to help children displaced by disasters to learn how to help younger children. This has been helpful in several disaster settings, including Afghan refugee camps in Pakistan.

Comfort Kits

These were originally developed by Dr. Tim Culbert to help children suffering from chronic pain. They were modified to help children who suffered in the tsunami in southern Thailand and in Haiti after the earthquake. The comfort kits include a pinwheel, a soft ball, six crayons, a small notebook, a bottle for blowing bubbles, and a finger puppet such as the Cat in the Hat. Accompanying instructions have been translated into Thai or Creole. The instructions explain how to color your feelings, how to breathe to relax with the bubbles or the pinwheel,how to use the puppet to help you feel better, how to relax all your muscles, and how to do imagery to feel better. The comfort kits were appealing to children in both Thailand and in Haiti where thousands were distributed.

18. Routines for Children

Children need to have some certainty and predictability in disaster situations. They experience terrible disruptions and losses when they leave familiar surroundings and become refugees. Those who have been separated from their family suffer the most. Provision of routines provides some stability and reduces anxiety. Routines for children should be planned as carefully as the distribution of food in disasters.

Routines for children may focus on feeding (especially important for the very young), play, school, religious or cultural activities, and work. Children and adolescents are often perceived as being in the way, as just hanging around, or as non-contributors in the aftermath of disasters. They can, in fact, help in a variety of tasks, such as caring for young unaccompanied minors, gathering wood, distributing water, working in gardens, making food, assisting in health clinics and making clothing. Adolescents can prepare entertainment programs for younger children. Depending on the culture, these may include pantomime, puppets, storytelling or musical programs.

There are often teachers, coaches, artists or musicians among displaced adults. When identified, they can be enlisted to help with organized programs for children. Adults should recognize the importance of role modeling in all situations, including disasters. They can provide surrogate parenting for children without parents. Adults should make sure that customary holidays are recognized and that festivities include children if culturally appropriate.

Schools can be conducted in most refugee settings, once the emergency phase has passed. Although books, chalkboards, paper and pencils may be unavailable, teaching can occur via voice, music, acting, use of leaves, stones or twigs to represent numbers for math problems, and other creative means. In warm climates classrooms can be organized outside. For example, in African refugee camps located in deserts, the outlines of classrooms have been marked with stones, and children sit within the stones.

Routines to be considered and established by relief workers include:

- Meals
- Bedtime
- School attendance
- Times for spontaneous play and imaginary play
- Religious/cultural events
- Sports
- Music
- Bathing
- Holidays and festivals

In summary, establishment of routines is reassuring to children in relief situations and should be a high priority in planning for them.

19. Media and Disasters

The realities of the 21st century have emphasized the important relationship between mass media and disasters. Mass media refers to means of mass communication, such as television, radio, newspapers, magazines, bulletins, periodical publications, audiovisual recordings, films or movies. The last century saw the explosion of global communication and mass media, from movies, to satellite communications, and ultimately the internet. This new century is seeing the development and improvement of many new forms of media, the mobile phone, podcasts, and other forms of mass communication, including social media, e.g. blogs, twitters, and Facebook.

The interaction of media and disasters is summarized by the statement published in the 2005 Workshop Summary on Disasters by the Institute of Medicine, "The media is the fastest, and in some cases, the only means to circulate important public health information to the public during a crisis; therefore, working with the media is critical to successful communication".

Media plays an important role in disaster relief and humanitarian assistance. Another definition for disaster is any health emergency situation making the front page or prime time news. If an emergency is not shown by the mass media, and is not in the news, there is no perception about its gravity or intensity.

For millions of people caught up in disasters, their survival depends on knowing what is happening and if they can expect help. Information is crucial and media is key to dispersing information. Disasters like Rwanda, Kosovo, the Indian Ocean Tsunami, Haiti earthquakes, and more recently the civil war in Syria, and typhoon Yolanda in the Philippines, have shown that media mobilizes attention to disasters. If this attention is properly channeled it can expedite humanitarian responses and save lives.

Media, Disasters and Children

After major disasters, TV and other media show scenes of devastation and destruction. It is impossible to keep children isolated from their surroundings. They see or hear about disasters and may be frightened. It is important to provide answers to children's questions. Honesty is essential, adults near children should provide simple and direct explanations, but it is not necessary to give more details than those asked by the children. Answers should be appropriate to the age of the child. Young children may confuse facts with their fantasies and fears. They may not realize that the same images are shown repeatedly by the media and may think the disaster is happening over and over again.

It is important that adults be sensitive to children's needs, recognizing that a child may be experiencing shock, fear and anxiety. Children who have had previous experiences in disasters may react more adversely to some media programs. For example, children who have lived through wars or earthquakes could have flashbacks. Children with pre-existing learning disabilities or emotional problems may have greater difficulties in coping with a disaster. Children's reactions to media may reflect their parents' reactions including fear, anger, dismay, or sadness.

Media can help children affected by disasters. Media can educate, give correct information, dispel rumors, request needed help, and create awareness of the special needs of children in disasters.

Child advocates can use the media to provide guidance on how to address children's needs in disasters, help children and families to cope with grief and losses, avoid exploitation of children and discuss the importance of addressing the psychosocial sequelae of disasters in children. It is extremely important to protect privacy of children when media is seeking to interview or photograph them. Relief workers should ask media to respect the dignity of children, their privacy, and their wishes in relation to media coverage. They should be prepared to report media representatives who breach the rights of children.

20.   Books and Reading for Children

Relief workers might think that focusing on getting books out and promoting reading time for young children after disasters should be delayed until medical facilities and treatment areas have been well established. As we have learned in the past decade in Indonesia, Haiti and after Hurricane Katrina, efforts to stabilize the emotional lives of children and provide comfort and understanding cannot be delayed. Books can help. Personal stories from relief workers in disasters have found books to be magic for sick and injured children and their families.

Through our growing experience with the Reach out and Read (ROR) program in the United States (www.reachoutandread.org), we have vastly increased our ability to find culturally appropriate books for all ages, starting from age 4–6 months, and to train parents, staff and volunteers, including older siblings, to help small children to interact with books. Child health professionals who have studied the ROR program have identified sources of inexpensive books appropriate for different ages (board books are important), the use of dialogic reading i.e. talking about books instead of just reading from them), and **how to** promote books for young children in their daily work.

Young children during times of disaster may sit as a little group of three or four on a barren cot, and there may be parents or relatives sitting beside them. This provides an ideal time to distribute books and to train parents and other adults on how to use books to comfort and encourage children. Even if parents cannot read, they can be taught how to use books to stimulate positive interactions with their children.

Noted Haitian-American author Edwidge Danticat's has written a children's book called Eight Days. Though this book describes the time spent by a seven year old trapped in his home after the 2010 earthquake, its dramatic illustrations can lift up its young readers. Ms Danticat says in her "Note from the Author" that in spite of unfathomable tragedy experienced, "Haiti's children still dream. They laugh. They live. They love." This is a perfect example of a book for young children experiencing tragedy, which is culturally appropriate and can contribute to healing.

After the tsunami disaster in southern Thailand Drs. Robert Needlman and Srivieng Pairojkul distributed books to hundreds of displaced children. Later, faculty from Khon Kaen University in northern Thailand established a mobile library which provided books to homes and schools for two years following the tsunami.

The desire to offer books to children in resource poor areas of the world has led to support for locally published, linguistically appropriate books for children around the world. ROR has made available their training videos for English speakers with internet access. Involvement of ROR advocates has led to locally published board books in Haiti, the Philippines and Lesotho in local languages.

What can Relief Workers Do?

They can bring appropriate books with them to disaster areas and demonstrate how they can be used. They can involve parents and other relatives of children or adolescents who benefit from useful volunteer work. They can seek sources of books in the countries where the disasters occur and create mobile libraries for displaced children. These mobile libraries do not necessarily require a car but may function with mopeds or bicycles or volunteers carrying baskets.

Ideal types of books for children at various stages:

Toddler – Board books that can be chewed, taken to bed and used as comfort objects. Recommended are photos of faces particularly those of local babies. One can point, count and sing. When possible, infants should be read to while sitting on the lap of the adult.

Preschool – Story books, especially local stories with familiar pictures of scenery, are recommended as are books about family, school and friends. Ask the child questions about the story and have the child tell his/her own version. Preschoolers also like books with rhyme.

Early school age – Continue to read aloud to children, although reading skills are taking off. Continue with numbers and letters and also hold the child while reading when possible. At this age children can start reading chapter books.

Pre adolescent – Children like books about adventure, animal fantasy stories, beginning poetry and books that include humor and/ or fantasy. The Magic Tree House series are enjoyed by many as are the Harry Potter series.

At this age and older good readers can read books on coping to younger children.

Adolescent – Good adolescent readers can be mobilized to read some of the healing and coping stories listed below either by themselves or to younger children. They might like to be distracted by fantasy books, series books, or comic books, especially those about teenagers.

Healing Books:

There are many books specifically written to help children to cope:

One specifically written for Haitian caregivers of children: *Thirty-Five Seconds (Trant Senk Segond)* by Dr. Marie Fonrose.

Others are:

- *A Terrible Thing Happened* by Holmes (lightweight with suggestions for caregivers)

- *The Boy who didn't want to be sad*, Goldblatt

- *101 Healing Stories for Kids and Teens: Using Metaphors in Therapy*, by George W. Burns

- *Harry, the Hypno-potamus: Metaphorical Tales for the Treatment of Children* vols 1 and 2 by Linda Thomson

- *Be the Boss of your Pain, Be the Boss of your Stress, and Be the Boss of Your Sleep* by Rebecca Kajander C.P.N.P. M.P.H. and Timothy Culbert M. Dr

These are examples of the types of books to help parents, relatives, and local volunteers provide comfort and pleasure to children after disasters. Most of the examples given would require English speakers. Appropriate books that are available in local languages should also be used.

Reference

Treating Traumatized Children, Rebecca Clay, American Psychological Association, July/August 2010, vol 41, No 7, Pp 36–38.

21.   Immunizations

Immunization protects against some of the most serious childhood diseases. In 1974 the WHO established the Expanded Program on Immunization (EPI) to ensure universal access to routinely recommended childhood vaccinations and six vaccine-preventable diseases were targeted: measles, diphtheria, pertussis, tetanus, polio, tuberculosis. While in 1974 less than 5% of the world's infants were fully immunized, by 2010 coverage for the 3rd dose of diphtheria-pertussis-tetanus (DPT) and measles-containing vaccine (MCV) had reached 85%. Nonetheless, in 2008, WHO estimated that 1.5 million deaths among children under five years were due to diseases that could have been prevented by routine vaccinations. This represents 17% of global total mortality in children under five years of age. Through immunization, children are protected against specific diseases and their dangerous complications. A child who is not immunized is more likely to become undernourished, disabled and die.

In emergency situations, the role of immunization must be prioritized in conjunction with the entire health situation. Relief workers should assess the pre disaster immunization status of displaced children. During the emergency phase, defined as that time during which the crude mortality rate (CMR) is higher than 1/10,000/day, the most common cause of disease and death is infection, often aggravated by malnutrition. Many of these early infections cannot be effectively prevented by immunization. Also, mass immunization programs consume a significant portion of available resources, which may be better utilized elsewhere during the emergency phase.

A recent 2012 report issued by the WHO's Strategic Advisory Group of Experts (SAGE) on Immunization highlights a lack of consensus regarding appropriate vaccination regimens during emergencies. Their literature review showed non-standardized criteria used by various organizations to plan and implement vaccination strategies. Nevertheless, there are a few themes that have generally been accepted regarding vaccination strategies during humanitarian crises. The only vaccines consistently recommended for mass immunization programs "immediately" during the emergency phase include measles, polio, and tetanus (for people with open wounds). Of the diseases that have epidemic potential, only three were recommended after the outset of an outbreak: hepatitis A, meningococcal meningitis, and yellow fever. In contrast, measles and polio have both been recommended for prevention and after the start of an outbreak. Notably, the documents that recommend polio vaccination for prevention during an emergency also address the potential threat to the ongoing eradication program (3). Interestingly, there are also ongoing discussions on whether preventive administration of the new meningococcal A conjugate vaccine for crises in the sub-Saharan African meningitis belt would be prudent as well. Routine tetanus, pertussis, and diphtheria vaccines are generally not recommended in emergency phase mass vaccination campaigns, although they should be initiated when conditions stabilize and the Expanded Program on Immunization (EPI) can be reinstated. Influenza and typhoid vaccines are usually not recommended at all during emergencies.

Measles is the most often recommended vaccination in the early phase of an emergency. It is a likely major cause of child mortality in humanitarian emergencies often aggravated by overcrowding in camps, preexisting malnutrition, and vitamin A deficiency. Many deaths attributed to diarrhea or pneumonia may be associated with measles, and case-fatality ratios of children in humanitarian emergencies have been estimated to be as high as 20–30% (4). The UNHCR Emergency Handbook in fact identifies measles immunization as the only essential immunization in the early stages of a crisis. Ideally, it should be distributed with vitamin A, as deficiencies are known to potentiate the severity of the disease. Humanitarian emergencies also often occur in populations with low herd immunity due to sociopolitical instability and disruption of routine vaccine programs and healthcare infrastructure. The balance between mass vaccination strategies in the setting of multiple urgent medical needs is understandably quite tenuous and dependent on multiple external factors as well such as cold chain supply, vaccine production supply, etc.

After the emergency phase has ended, an immunization program should be established as an integral part of the long-term health program. Each situation must be evaluated to determine which diseases take priority, what is the magnitude of the problem and what are the vaccination capabilities. Due to the substantial resources required, immunization should be targeted against the diseases that have the highest potential to cause morbidity and mortality. In order to determine the size of the group at risk for developing disease, the degree of existing immunity must be determined. Existing immunity may be secondary to previous exposure or prior immunization. Efforts should be made to identify groups who are at higher risk of disease, such as those who are malnourished, immunocompromised or with close contact to affected individuals.

The following table adapted from the 2012 WHO's SAGE Report lists recommendations on vaccine-preventable diseases in emergency situations and the organizations that support the recommendation.

Vaccine-Preventable Disease / Vaccine	Supporting Organization	Summary of Recommendations	Crisis conditions for Risk Factors for Disease	Recommended Timing of Vaccination Relative to Emergency Onset
Cholera (Oral Cholera Vaccine)	WHO,	The use of OCV in emergencies continues to be under dispute.	Overcrowding, inadequate sanitation facilities and contamination of water sources, poor hygiene conditions (personal, domestic and environmental), poor nutritional status and low immunity prior to the infection8	No recommendation relative to the phase of emergency. Before a cholera outbreak has been declared.
	UNHCR,	The UNHCR and UNICEF recommend seeking expert advice and considering the use of OCV under the most recent evidence-based guidelines.		
	UNICEF	The use of OCV should be assessed in light of other public health priorities and other priority interventions. It is not recommended for use after the start of an epidemic. Risk assessment and decision making tool has been developed and requires field validation. Under some circumstances, for example in Haiti after the 2010 earthquake, it was not recommended, and the CDC does not recommend OCV for evacuees following a disaster.		
	IFRC	Cholera vaccine may be considered preventively, in a stable, endemic environment, but is of limited use once an epidemic has begun. High risk populations may be targeted for pre-emptive use.		
	IAP			
	US CDC			
Hemophilus influenza type b (Hib) and S. pneumonia (PCV)		Recommended for use in the prevention of severe bacterial infections, but these vaccines not often available in emergencies.		Early phase of displacement.
Hepatitis A	Various	In case of an outbreak, targeted vaccination with Hep A for populations at risk and may be considered for contacts. Not recommended for mass immunization, and may be considered for persons at high risk, i.e. those involved in management of drinking water, waste water, or sewage. Hep A not routinely recommended after disasters, as a result of evacuation due to natural disaster alone or in the drought and famine in the Horn of Africa.	Lack of water, sanitation and hygiene	Mainly recommended in case of outbreak

Vaccine-Preventable Disease / Vaccine	Supporting Organization	Summary of Recommendations	Crisis conditions for Risk Factors for Disease	Recommended Timing of Vaccination Relative to Emergency Onset
Hepatitis B		No indication for mass vaccination with Hep B vaccine in emergency generally, however some indication for vaccination for those handling dead bodies who may be more at risk of blood borne infections.	Unsafe injection practices, blood transfusion, injection drug use, occurrence of mass casualties in endemic countries, workers with exposure to with dead bodies	Not a general concern during the acute phase.
Influenza	US CDC	Recommended for evacuees in crowded group settings after a natural disaster (if cannot prove to have recently received it). Not proven to be useful post-earthquake, beyond routine selective usage.	Crowded group setting	Not stated.
	WHO	Seasonal influenza vaccine is not recommended for an outbreak of a novel influenza virus in displaced populations, as there will likely not be sufficient quantities to cover the global population.		
Measles (MCV, MMR)	WHO	Measles immunization is a priority health intervention in emergencies, and may be considered the only essential immunization in the early stages of an emergency.	Displacement, severe food shortage, malnutrition, overcrowding, low measles vaccine coverage, lack of essentials for life	During the immediate 6–8 weeks of a crisis, or as soon as possible, and should not await a single case.
	UNICEF	Should be administered to all children 6 months through 15 years of age, and at minimum to all children aged 6–59 months. An opportunity for second dose should be given to those immunized prior to 9 months of age, once they reach 9 months, with a minimum of one month between doses. In some cases groups older than 15 should be considered in the target age, based on risk assessment.		
	UNHCR	Where resources are limited, priority groups are children <5 and those at high risk (i.e. malnourished). Measles morbidity and mortality in malnourished children is easily preventable with vaccination.		
	IFRC	Non-selective approach with at least 90% coverage is required.		
	US CDC	Recommended coupling with Vitamin A supplementation to reduce complications of measles.		
	SPHERE	The US CDC recommends in conditions of displacement to crowded group settings after disaster, evacuees should be given MMR, unless proof of coverage is provided.		
	Various organizations	Phased approach to implementation of interventions, based on a needs assessment. Provide simultaneous vaccination campaigns in the refugee populations and the surrounding host community.		

Vaccine-Preventable Disease / Vaccine	Supporting Organization	Summary of Recommendations	Crisis conditions for Risk Factors for Disease	Recommended Timing of Vaccination Relative to Emergency Onset
Meningococcal	WHO,	Meningitis is one of the major vaccines used in complex emergencies. Meningitis vaccine offers effective control of epidemics. Should be implemented only after expert advice, when surveys suggest necessity, and only at the outset of an outbreak to children >2 y old.	Overcrowding in areas where disease is endemic	At outset of an outbreak
Meningitis	UNHCR, IFRC, IAP		Local dry season seasonal pattern)	
Pertussis	WHO	Vaccination in response to a pertussis outbreak are generally avoided due to theoretical concerns regarding adverse events in adolescents and adults when given the whole cell DTP vaccine.	Crowding, malnutrition, coinfection with other illness (HIV, malaria, TB, etc.)	Not applicable.
Polio	WHO,	Polio transmission is a threat to eradication programs, and is linked to poor water and sanitation. In the Horn of Africa, during drought and famine, recommend OPV to all children <5 yrs in conjunction with measles and vitamin A supplementation	Famine, malnutrition, crowded refugee camps, low pre-existing vaccine coverage, conflict, floods	Immediately after onset of emergency, or at the outset of an outbreak.
	IFRC	At the outset of an outbreak, all children should receive at least 1 dose, with a second round of mass vaccination after 30 days. Vaccination is recommended with bivalent vaccine rather than trivalent vaccine.		
Rabies	CDC	For post-exposure prophylaxis only	Exposure to rabies	Not specifically related to emergency
Tetanus (TT; Td)	UNICEF;	For pregnant women and women of child-bearing age.	Unhygienic conditions, sustainment of injury and wounds with potential for contamination	Early stages of emergency and in post-emergency stage.
	UNHCR, IFRC	In post-emergency, EPI should include either TT or Td, at least 2 doses.		
		For open wounds: Mass tetanus vaccination not recommended. Targeted active and passive vaccination to individuals who sustain open wounds or are involved with clean up after a disaster. Not necessary to give TT or tetanus immunoglobulin (TIG) to patients who have had complete series and a booster within the last 10 years. Immediate provision of Td vaccine and tetanus anti-toxin to persons injured during earthquake and those undergoing emergency surgeries.		

As discussed above, once conditions stabilize in an emergency situation, it is imperative that routine immunization programs such as the Expanded Program on Immunization be reinstituted. The routine immunization schedule in most countries is composed of six preventable diseases: measles, diphtheria, pertussis, tetanus, polio, and tuberculosis. Table 1 provides a brief description about the key characteristics of these diseases. It is also worth noting that some countries also include Hemophilus influenza type B, Hepatitis B, and Yellow Fever in their immunization schedules. Women of childbearing age should also be administered tetanus toxoid vaccine to prevent neonatal tetanus. Routine vitamin A distribution is often integrated into the national EPI program and targets children under 5 years as well as postnatal mothers. Tables 2–4 provide general guidelines established by the WHO.

Table 1: Characteristics of Major Vaccine Preventable Illnesses

Measles	Highly contagious respiratory disease with symptoms of rash, high fever, cough, runny nose, red watery eyes, lasting approximately one week. Common complications include ear infections and pneumonia, whereas more rare complications include encephalitis, deafness, or mental retardation
Diphtheria	Highly contagious respiratory disease with gradual onset of sore throat, low grade fever, and development of membrane in the throat which may interfere with swallowing or breathing
Pertussis	Highly contagious respiratory disease spread through intense coughing in 3 clinical stages: 1) catarrhal stage (1–2 weeks): gradually increasing cough, runny nose, fever, and decreased appetite; 2) paroxysmal (2–4 weeks): paroxysms of coughing (with a whoop) triggered by eating, drinking, talking, and crying, can be associated with blue spells, vomiting, and hypoxia. Complications include bronchopneumonia, encephalitis, and neurologic sequelae mostly related to episodes of hypoxia
Polio	Transmitted through fecal-oral transmission (poor hand-washing, or water contamination). Symptoms include fever, sore throat, nausea, headaches, abdominal pain, neck and back pain. Can lead to eventual paralysis and death.
Tetanus	Neurologic disease caused by bacteria that enter the body through a break in the skin (e.g. a puncture wound). Early symptoms include headache, irritability, jaw and neck stiffness, and later develop into severe muscular spasms in the jaw, neck, arms, legs, back, and abdomen. Frequently occurs in the neonatal form in low and middle income countries due to lack of maternal immunization.
Tuberculosis	Highly infectious respiratory disease which can be active or latent. Symptoms include weight loss, fevers, night sweats, cough productive of mucus or blood, chest pain, and swollen lymph nodes.

Table 2: Recommended EPI Schedule for routine immunization (WHO)

New Visit	Diseases	Age
BCG	Tuberculosis	At birth
DPT	Diphtheria, Pertussis, Tetanus	6, 10, 14 weeks
OPV	Polio	At birth, 6, 10, 14 weeks
Measles	Measles	9 months

Table 3: Recommended Schedule for Tetanus Toxoid Administration (WHO)

Dose	Time for administration	Duration of protection
TT1	At first contact	No protection
TT2	4 weeks after TT1	Three years
TT3	At least 6 months after TT2	Five years
TT4	At least 1 year after TT3	Ten years
TT5	At least 1 year after TT4	For thirty years

Table 4: Recommended schedule for Vitamin A Distribution

Age group	Dosage	Frequency
<6 months	50,000 IU	6, 10, 14 weeks
6–12 months	100,000 IU	Every 4–6 months
>= 12 months	200,000 IU	Every 4–6 months
Mother	400,000 IU	<=6–8 weeks postpartum

There are very few contraindications for vaccination. According to the WHO, "routine vaccinations should be administered unless the child's condition makes hospitalization necessary." Vaccination of immunocompromised children is frequently avoided. However, in countries where the chance of measles and polio infection is high, the risk of vaccination must be carefully weighed against the risk of acquiring disease. At present, BCG is contraindicated in children presenting with clinical signs of AIDS; all other immunizations are indicated. Fear of interruption of the vaccine schedule should not preclude initiation of immunization programs. Interruptions will not lead to the need to repeat the entire schedule. Malnutrition is not a contraindication for vaccination.

All immunization programs must be continually evaluated. Careful records should be kept to determine the number of vaccines given, the number of children immunized and the preservation of the cold chain. The cold chain requires that vaccines be kept continuously refrigerated, even in transit, in order to maintain potency. Immunization effectiveness can be measured through a comparison of the incidence of disease in children immunized vs. children not immunized. In order to facilitate evaluation and to best serve the children, all children should be given an immunization record.

Efforts to support lactating women are a key component of any immunization program. The immunity conferred to infants through breastfeeding should not be underestimated. Human milk protects and promotes infant health by augmenting the child's immature immune system.

VACCINE INJECTION TECHNIQUE

The route and site of vaccine injection affect vaccine efficacy. Diphtheria, tetanus and pertussis vaccines should be administered intramuscularly. Inactivated polio vaccine (IPV), meningococcal and measles vaccines should be injected subcutaneously. Injection technique and needle length are both important to proper vaccine delivery.

Injectable vaccines should be administered in a site as free as possible from the risk of local neural, vascular or tissue injury. Preferred sites include the anterolateral aspect of the upper thigh and deltoid area of the upper arm. These sites are good for vaccines administered either subcutaneously or intramuscularly. The WHO technique for intramuscular injection involves stretching the skin flat between the finger and thumb, and pushing the needle down at a 90-degree angle through the skin. This technique should be used in combination with a 16 mm (5/8-inch) needle for effective intramuscular delivery.

VACCINE HANDLING AND STORAGE

Improper vaccine storage conditions can lead to vaccine failures. Certain vaccines, such as oral polio and measles, are very sensitive to increased temperature. Others vaccines are sensitive to freezing. The latter include diphtheria, tetanus, pertussis and IPV. Recommendations for the handling and storage of vaccines are summarized in the package insert for each product. All personnel involved in vaccine handling must be familiar with the standard storage procedures to minimize vaccine failure.

WHO publications and the American Academy of Pediatrics Red Book contain detailed guidelines regarding the personnel, equipment and procedures needed to run an effective immunization program.

22.   Medical Issues

Dr. Jordana Hikri

The medical needs of children in disasters vary depending on the area of the world, their prior immunizations, the season and the level of sanitation. In general, the primary medical risks relate to malnutrition and to infectious diseases. In many situations children are at risk for injuries related to unexploded ordnance, traffic accidents, dog bites, drowning, physical abuse and/or flying debris (as in an earthquake or tornado). Some basic resource books that are helpful in addressing pediatric medical needs are listed in the last chapter of this manual.

Whether or not the immediate medical needs of children can be met depends on the state of the local medical system prior to the disaster and/or how the local medical system is itself affected directly by the disaster. For example, consider the devastating earthquake that struck Haiti in 2010. At that time, there were eleven hospitals in the capital city, Port-au-Prince. At least eight of these were damaged or destroyed by the earthquake, leaving the remaining institutions overwhelmed. In contrast, when earthquakes of similar magnitude struck Tokyo in 2009 and Chile in 2010, the damage to the healthcare system (and the resultant loss of life) was far less, in part owing to better medical infrastructure and a more established medical system.

Children's unique physiology impacts their outcome in a disaster. For example, children's higher respiratory rate and minute volume increases their exposure to inhaled infectious and chemical agents. Their increased metabolic rate results in greater relative exposure to radiation and chemical agents. In addition, these agents often settle low to the ground, thus affecting children more so than adults. Children are at increased risk of dehydration and hypothermia/hyperthermia. Their higher surface-to-volume ratio makes them more prone to absorbable toxins. Younger children, and those with physical or intellectual disabilities, are also less able to physically remove themselves from harm's way, or to anticipate danger.

In addition, in many disaster situations children are left without appropriate adult supervision and protection. This reality increases their risk for injuries (including from "non-disaster" sources such as traffic accidents, dog bites, and drowning), as well as their risk of falling victim to physical or sexual abuse. The following is an overview of the myriad medical issues facing children in disasters, along with some basic interventions. Additional resources are listed in the last chapter of this manual.

TRIAGE AND PATIENT FLOW

In a disaster situation, it may seem impossible to keep up with the demand of seeing so many sick children every day. Therefore, triage skills are an essential part of training for humanitarian emergencies. The triage system should quickly identify those patients who require emergent care (as available, given your resources), those who require rapid transfer to escalated care, and those who can wait. Such a system requires careful planning and trained personnel. However, even in the "clinic" situation, it is essential that an experienced person scan the waiting children to select those who are sickest to be examined first. If you have few health professionals available, train as many laypeople as possible to assist with tasks such as checking heights/weights/vital signs, cleaning the examination area, counting out pills, etc.

Once you have a clinic management system, and if there are large numbers of children to be examined, move yourself as little as possible. Let the child be brought to you, on the caretaker's lap or on a table in front of you. Make an effort to learn some key greetings and medical phrases, as the need for interpretation greatly slows the process. Remember, in many situations, the examiner will hear the same questions—and the same answers—many times a day!

THINGS TO KEEP IN MIND

Nutrition and Hydration

* **Clean drinking water must be a priority.**

Clean drinking water helps to prevent epidemics of infectious disease, which so often occur after disasters—for example, the cholera in Haiti after the 2010 earthquake. The fecal-oral route most often spreads infection through uprooted populations. As such, providing clean drinking water and basic sanitation is considered one of WHO's

Essential Emergency Relief Measures. See the chapter on Water and Sanitation for recommended methods of water purification and sanitation.

* Ready-made packets of oral rehydration-therapy (ORT) powder or high protein re-feeding mixtures may be unavailable.

Be prepared to improvise these treatments using local ingredients (see the end of this chapter for a basic ORT recipe). In NW Pakistan, for example, the carbohydrate comes from wheat flour, whereas in NW China it is composed of millet and sugar.

* Reliable measuring tools are helpful.

If you don't have them, request them or improvise. You can make a height/length board out of smooth wood and a known standard. A Broselow Tape can help estimate weights if a scale is not available. There has recently been a study showing that the 2D and 3D MercyTAPE is more reliable than the Broselow Tape. 25 kilogram hanging Salter scales should be requested. If possible children should be suspended in a basket for weighing, rather than the uncomfortable hanging pants or slings.

* Growth charts are for the whole world.

An unfortunate rationalization for the acceptance of stunting as "normal" is the common belief that WHO growth charts are correct for Western populations only. There are a few exceptions, but in general, children from all ethnic groups should fall within the new standards developed by WHO (revised as of 2006).

Infectious Diseases

* The milieu of a disaster makes children more susceptible to infectious disease.

Anxiety, depression, malnutrition, poor sanitation and exposure to new organisms all increase the likelihood that children will get sick. While fecal-oral diseases are often mentioned, significant spread of respiratory illnesses can also occur following a disaster, especially when survivors are forced to live together in close quarters. Respiratory transmission may be enhanced by inhalation of respiratory irritants, such as smoke from open fires. In addition, vector-borne infections often increase following disasters, especially when there is a great deal of standing water—as might occur following a flood or a tsunami.

* **Prevention should be concurrent with acute care.**

Re-establishment of primary care, as well as disease surveillance, are among WHO's Essential Emergency Relief Measures. If you treat many children with the same infectious disease, ask about immediate interventions that can prevent additional cases (e.g. sanitation, vaccinations). To assist with surveillance, one should ideally keep a patient log with (at minimum) age, sex, and diagnosis. Regularly review this log and share your findings with any public health officials in the area.

Provide measles immunization and vitamin A supplementation

Another one of WHO's Essential Emergency Relief Measures, measles vaccination is the only vaccine routinely considered to be a post-disaster preventative intervention. This is due to the fact that among crowded, malnourished populations, measles is a major source of mortality. Vaccination should begin before measles cases are reported. Recall that following 10–12 days of incubation there is a 2–4 day prodrome of fever, cough, coryza, conjunctivitis, and Koplik spots. Isolation is ineffective since the disease is most contagious during the prodromal phase. Only later does the characteristic maculopapular descending rash appear.

Complications of measles include rapid weight loss, pneumonia, croup, otitis media, diarrhea, immune suppression and blindness. Vitamin A deficiency is common and increases measles-related mortality—therefore supplementation is recommended for vulnerable exposed populations. The recommended dose is 50,000 IU for infants under 6 months, 100,000 IU for infants 6–12 months, and 200,000 IU for children over 12 months. All of these should be followed by another identical dose given 24 hours later. See the Chapter on Immunizations for more information regarding the recommended distribution and timing of measles vaccination and vitamin A supplementation.

* Malaria Pearls

Malaria causes 1–2 million deaths annually, mostly in children under age five. It is an endemic disease in many parts of the world, and in those areas any fever should be considered malaria until proven otherwise. When providing medical care in a disaster, it is crucial to understand the local patterns of species prevalence and drug resistance. Keep in mind that with uprooted populations, naïve individuals may be exposed to new stains of malaria. When clinical history and presentation suggest malaria, begin treatment immediately—as even patients with cerebral malaria can initially present with negative smears.

* Treatment of intestinal parasites is not a priority in an acutely ill child.

Although it is still important to inquire about signs and symptoms of parasitic infection, the benefit of antihelminthics and purges for intestinal parasites is generally not worth the risks of toxicity and bowel obstruction or volvulus. Use these drugs after the child's general status has improved.

* Breast is best

The AAP recommends that clinicians encourage breast-feeding whenever possible in disaster situations. Doing so provides infants with ideal nutrition and immunity advantages, while avoiding food-and-water-associated infections. Mothers, however, may require significant support to continue (or re-establish) breastfeeding. Of note, malnourished mothers can still provide quality breast milk.

If maternal breastfeeding is not possible, HIV-negative donor milk should be used. If this is not available, then ready-to-feed formula should be given. Powder formulas are a last resort. Regarding the risk of HIV transmission, WHO recommends offering HIV testing to women. If they decline or if testing is unavailable, breastfeeding is recommended. If a woman is HIV-positive, she requires individual risk counseling regarding options and associated risks. See the Chapter on Nutrition for more information.

Medications and Supplies

* Supportive care in a pediatric hospital is not assured.

Hospitals may not have adequate staff to tend intravenous lines, give medications on schedule, feed ill children, etc. If parents are not available to provide supplemental care, special arrangements must be made for ill children.

* Malnutrition affects pharmacokinetics in children.

Whether by affecting absorption, half-life, or metabolism, protein-energy malnutrition (PEM) has a significant effect on the pharmacokinetics of certain medications, especially those metabolized by the liver. Best efforts should be made to choose medications and dosages accordingly. For example, acetaminophen is not recommended in PEM because it causes increased absorption and decreased clearance.

* Many drugs have negative side effects with respect to nutrition.

Many of our most commonly-used medications have a negative impact on children's nutritional status. For example, consider the many medications that can cause anorexia, nausea/vomiting, malabsorption, diarrhea, deranged vitamin metabolism, etc. These side effects may become significant in a child whose nutrition/hydration status is borderline.

* Drugs stored under incorrect conditions may lose potency.

The majority of medications stored under ambient conditions in climates with high heat and humidity will not be effective after two to three months. Keep in mind that refrigeration may not be available or reliable. If a child is not responding to a medication, consider whether or not the medication has lost potency or whether it might be a fake medication or whether the microbial agent is resistant to the drug.

* Blankets and clothing are part of treatment.

When the environment is cold, calories are burned to maintain body temperature. Malnourished and young children die from exposure in cool climates.

* **Disposable equipment is reused.**

Syringes, IV tubing and gloves are often reused in disaster situations, with increased risk for transmission of diseases such as HIV and Hepatitis B. Re-sterilization of disposable equipment is often not possible.

* **Remember to bring your own examining equipment.**

Child health practitioners who are preparing to help in a disaster should try to bring with them as much equipment as possible. In general, bring your own stethoscope, otoscope and ophthalmoscope, at a minimum. It is wise to bring a pediatric BP cuff, percussion hammer, small emergency medication kit, and plenty of gloves. Other items to consider:

* **Airway Management/Breathing**

Tongue blades, suction (portable, battery-powered) and catheters, face masks (infant, child, adult) for assisted ventilation, self-inflating bags (250 cc, 500 cc, and 1000 cc reservoir)

* **For intubation**

Laryngoscope handle, extra batteries and laryngoscope bulbs, assorted blades and endotracheal tubes, laryngeal mask airways, stylets, ET CO_2 analyzer, and adhesive tape to secure ET tubes

* **Circulation/Intravascular Access or Fluid Management**

Assorted IV catheters and butterfly needles, intraosseous needles or Eazy IO device, boards, tape, pediatric drip chambers and tubing, IV fluids

Medications: epinephrine, atropine, sodium bicarbonate, calcium chloride, lidocaine, D25, D10

* Miscellaneous

- Broselow tape, 2D or 3D MercyTAPE, assorted nasogastric tubes, splints and gauze padding, blankets, warm water source, portable showers for decontamination, radiant heat lamps, Geiger counter (if suspicion of radioactive contamination), additional personal protective equipment (PPE), surgical equipment for incision and drainage of wounds and laceration repairs, headlamps with replacement batteries, scissors, plaster for casting (not fiberglass, which can be difficult to remove)

- Pain\ Sedation medications: ibuprofen, acetaminophen, ketamine, morphine, ketorolac, numbing creams, distracting tools such as Buzzy Bee, pinwheels, toys etc.

- Other potential medications: albuterol, Keflex, Ancef, ceftriaxone, diazepam, multivitamins, ferrous sulfate

* Monitoring Equipment

Sphygmomanometer/ Blood pressure cuffs (premature, infant, child, adult), portable monitor/defibrillator (with settings < 10), pediatric defibrillation paddles, pediatric electrocardiogram (ECG) skin electrode contacts (peel and stick), pulse oximeter with sensors, serum glucose monitoring device, urinalysis strips.

Cross-cultural issues

Traditional Medicine

In the United States, about a third of families regularly use complementary and alternative medical treatments (CAM). In the less industrialized world, roughly eighty per cent of health care is provided through traditional means. CAM includes herbal remedies, healing ceremonies, acupuncture, moxibustion, and more.

In disaster situations, families may bring traditional medication with them, and traditional healers are often very popular. Keep in mind that local practitioners often know a lot about treating children in their environment. Ask them for advice and work with them. This includes showing them respect and engaging them in health projects.

In addition, recognize that cross-cultural issues can affect medical care. If you do not know, ask questions about cultural taboos related to examinations, medications, foods, etc. In addition, if possible, it is important to learn about plant-derived traditional treatments, as there may be dangerous interactions between herbal treatments and prescribed medications. Always inquire if your patient has used any traditional remedies prior to choosing your therapy.

Interpreters vary in ability.

Many interpreters who offer their services in urgent situations have no medical background. In addition, if the social status of the interpreter is too different from that of the patient—or on the other hand, if the interpreter is overly familiar—it may be difficult to obtain accurate information. If possible, train interpreters in basic medical terminology, objective interpretation skills, confidentiality, etc.

Children, in general, fear strangers who offer medical care.

In some cultures, children do not express their fear as directly as do many Western children. Recognize that fear may be present, and may leave a negative impression that lasts a lifetime. In spite of the urgency and chaos, do whatever you can to mitigate the child's fear. Carry a few toys, play with the child, and examine the child in the parents' arms. Special consideration should be given to pain control, especially when required to perform invasive procedures. In addition to numbing/cooling, do not discount the benefits of distraction, such as Buzzy Bee, pinwheels (which help to focus breathing), culturally appropriate music, or other toys.

Consider the psychosocial element.

In addition to the usual history, find out how long it has been since the children left their home. Did they witness or experience violence? Did they lose a family member? If the children are able to speak, are they speaking normally since the disaster? Who is the usual caretaker? Keep in mind that it may be a sibling. Are the parents or caretakers ill?

IMCI

IMCI is a program developed by WHO that aims to help prevent and treat medical problems which lack child health specialists and sophisticated diagnostic tools. The program focuses on the major causes of childhood mortality: diarrhea, acute respiratory infections, malnutrition, malaria, and measles.

An IMCI assessment begins by looking for specific "danger signs": seizures, lethargy or unconsciousness, inability to drink/breastfeed, or persistent vomiting. Any child with even one danger sign should be sent to a hospital. Next, sick children are assessed for a select number of key symptoms: cough or difficulty breathing, diarrhea, fever, or ear problems. Nutrition and immunization status, anemia, and other issues are explored. Finally, using the IMCI protocol, a color-coded assessment is made. ORANGE requires urgent referral to an inpatient healthcare facility. YELLOW requires treatment at an outpatient healthcare facility. GREEN patients can be managed at home. Major components of IMCI are specific treatment protocols, maternal education, and provisions for follow-up care. Of note, IMCI does not address complicated differential diagnoses, chronic diseases, uncommon illnesses, or trauma.

Most of the IMCI documents are easily accessible on line; e.g. the manual Management of the Child with a Serious Infection or Severe Malnutrition: Guidelines for care at the First Referral Level in Developing Countries has detailed information for the management of sick children following the IMCI guidelines. (See URL in Resources)

SIGNS AND SYMPTOMS

This section represents useful observations collected through our years of experience in the field. Acute signs and symptoms may represent tropical, infectious or parasitic diseases in children. While one often lacks laboratory and radiological tools to facilitate diagnoses, it is helpful to think of both usual and unusual differential diagnoses that might explain signs and symptoms in a sick child.

* **Sign or symptom • Think of:**

- Buboes (large lymph nodes) • Plague.

- Cardiac failure • Beriberi, Chagas disease, diphtheria, Lassa fever, nematode myocarditis, pericardial amebiasis, unrecognized congenital heart disease.

- Coma, semicoma • Cerebral malaria, TB meningitis, sleeping sickness (trypanosomiasis).

- Cough, Tachypnea • Melioidosis, tuberculosis, hydatid lung cyst, pulmonary phase of nematode migration.

- Conjunctival injection • Marburg and Ebola virus disease, measles.

- Diarrhea, dehydration • Malaria, melioidosis.

- Fever of unknown origin • Malaria, typhoid, tick fever, rabies, Lassa fever, trypanosomiasis, dengue.

- Edema (Palpebral) • Chagas disease.

- Erythema Nodosum • Leprosy.

- Gray Skin • Leishmaniasis (kala azar).

- Hallucinations • Malaria, Japanese B encephalitis, rabies, Lassa fever, Venezuelan equine encephalitis.

- Headache with paresthesias • Eosinophilic meningitis.

- Hematuria • Schistosomiasis, bladder stone, tuberculosis.

- Hepatomegaly • Ameboma, kala azar, flukes, hepatitis

- Intestinal obstruction • Nematode bolus, amebiasis.

- Iritis, keratitis • Onchocerciasis.

- Jaundice • Malaria, typhoid, schistosomiasis, kala azar.

- Malnutrition • Tuberculosis, AIDS, kala azar.

- Nasal obstruction • Myiasis.

- Nephrotic syndrome • Malaria, leprosy.

- Palpebral edema • Chagas' disease.

- Paralyses • Polio, schistosomiasis, konzo (cyanide poisoning via cassava), tuberculosis.

- Petechiae, purpura • Dengue shock syndrome, Korean hemorrhagic fever, Ebola fever, typhus.

- Pneumonia • Melioidosis, tuberculosis.

- Rash • Measles, dengue, vitamin deficiencies, scabies.

- Splenomegaly • Kala azar, malaria, typhoid.

- Seizures • Tetanus, cysticercosis, malaria, rabies, TB meningitis, eosinophilic meningoencephalitis, Japanese B encephalitis.

- Shock syndrome • Dengue, intestinal perforation due to typhoid, Ebola fever, malaria.

- Skin nodules/ulcers • Onchocerciasis, leprosy, anthrax, melioidosis, typhus, cutaneous leishmaniasis, gnathostomiasis, dracontiasis.

- Stroke • Cysticercosis, Sickle cell disease.

- Transient swellings • Filiariasis (loa loa).

DIFFERENTIAL DIAGNOSES

Regardless of the area of the world, the following conditions may explain observed signs and symptoms. Careful history may help to include or exclude some of these entities:

- AIDS.
- Acute appendicitis.
- Bacterial meningitis.
- Cardiac failure.
- Cat scratch disease.
- Collagen-vascular diseases such as rheumatoid arthritis.
- Infectious hepatitis, A, B, C, E.
- Malignancies.
- Metabolic diseases such as hypothyroidism or diabetes.
- Micronutrient deficiencies, e.g. beriberi.
- Pertussis.
- Physical or sexual abuse.
- Pneumonia.
- Poisoning.
- Rabies.
- Roseola.
- Scabies.
- Salmonellosis.
- Shigella dysentery.
- Streptococcal Pharyngitis.
- Syphilis.
- Tetanus.
- Toxic reaction to medications.
- Tuberculosis.
- Urinary tract infections.

INFECTIOUS DIARRHEAL DISEASES

Diarrheal diseases (and resultant dehydration) are major causes of morbidity and mortality in the disaster setting. The following is a brief overview of some of the more common etiologies of infectious diarrhea, and some recommendations regarding therapy.

It is helpful to divide diarrhea into three categories: acute watery diarrhea, acute bloody diarrhea or dysentery, and persistent diarrhea (lasting more than 14 days). Each category tends to have specific causal agents, health implications, and recommendations for treatment.

Acute Watery Diarrhea

Acute watery diarrhea is most often caused by viruses including rotavirus and norwalk-like virus, or by bacteria such as enterotoxigenic Escherichia coli (ETEC), Vibrio cholerae, Staphylococcus aureus, Clostridium difficile, Giardia, and cryptosporidia. Usually, acute watery diarrhea is a self-limited condition and treatment is supportive. With few exceptions, antibiotics are not only not required to treat acute watery diarrhea, but may potentially prolong the disease by interfering with the repopulation of normal gut flora. Similarly, antidiarrheal and antiemetic medications reduce gut motility and prolong pathogen exposure, and therefore are not recommended. After providing appropriate rehydration, encourage patients to resume their normal diet. Fasting or avoiding lactose provides no benefits, and reduced oral consumption reduces gut motility and the cellular turnover needed for healing.

Symptoms of Vibrio cholerae include painless, afebrile, "rice-water" diarrhea that can rapidly progress to electrolyte derangement and shock. Cholera survives independently for days, spreads rapidly, and is a true public health emergency. The index case of suspected cholera should be cultured for sensitivities, but subsequent cases can be diagnosed clinically. Treatment includes rehydration, and appropriate antibiotics.

Acute Bloody Diarrhea

Acute bloody diarrhea (or dysentery) is usually caused by more invasive enteric agents such as Shigella, Entamoeba histolytica,

Campylobacter sp, invasive Escherichia coli, Salmonella, aeromonas organisms, C. difficile, and Yersinia sp. These infections tend to cause more significant morbidity and mortality, including malnutrition, severe dehydration, and sepsis. Therefore, the Integrated Management of Childhood Illness (IMCI) program recommends antibiotics for any child with dysentery. Antibiotic therapy aims to improve clinical symptoms and to decrease fecal shedding of the pathogen. After appropriate rehydration, treat for 5 days with an anti-Shigella agent (as the majority of childhood dysentery is caused by Shigella). Shigella resistance patterns vary, so be aware of local sensitivities. Ideally, obtain a stool culture prior to treatment so that antibiotics can be tailored appropriately. If there is no clinical improvement after 48 hours of antibiotics, refer the child to more specialized care. Of note, any bloody diarrhea in a child under 2 months requires urgent referral, as well.

Certain regions have a higher incidence of shiga toxin-producing enterohemorrhagic E. Coli (EHEC), which can cause hemolytic-uremic syndrome (HUS). Antibiotics can precipitate or worsen renal failure in HUS. Therefore, when treating bloody diarrhea in these areas, if stool cultures are available, it is recommended to observe them for 48 hours. This allows the practitioner to choose appropriate antibiotics, or to avoid antibiotics if the patient is found to have EHEC.

In addition to bacteria, the protozoan Entamoeba histolytica can also cause bloody diarrhea. Infections usually progress gradually (over 3–4 weeks), and children may be less ill-appearing than those with bacterial dysentery. Entamoeba histolytica infections are sometimes associated with fever, abdominal pain, intermittent diarrhea/constipation, and hepatomegaly. Possible sequelae include toxic megacolon, fulminant colitis, bowel perforation, and liver abscess. When amoebic infection is suspected (either due to microscopic stool analysis, or two failed courses of antibiotics), treat with metronidazole at 30 mg/kg/day for 5–10 days.

Persistent Diarrhea

Children with persistent diarrhea (lasting more than 14 days) are at increased risk of morbidity and mortality. If there are any signs of dehydration, the child should be rehydrated and referred to a hospital. Any infant under two months with more than 7 days of diarrhea should also be referred.

For those children who appear well-hydrated upon presentation, the main goal of therapy should be to optimize nutrition and minimize gut irritation, in order to allow for recovery. To that end, parents should limit animal milk and other lactose-containing foods to no more than 50 mL/kg/day. Encourage breast-feeding, when possible. If the child is over six months, give small frequent feeds of appropriate complementary foods. No specific antibiotic therapy is recommended, unless further investigation reveals an identified causal agent.

One such agent is the protozoan Giardia. Giardiasis tends to cause a sub-acute, afebrile illness consisting of non-bloody, foul-selling, greasy diarrhea associated with cramps, abdominal pain

Rehydration

The mainstay of therapy in all types of diarrhea is to provide rehydration. Oral Rehydration Therapy (ORT) is the most safe and efficacious means of preventing deaths from diarrhea-related dehydration. In brief, ORT takes advantage of active sodium-glucose co-transport in the gut cell wall (as diarrhea tends to impair passive sodium absorption). As such, ORT solutions are usually composed of equimolar amounts of both salt and sugar (or starch). Since ORT relies on physiologic mechanisms, it is safe to use in all types of dehydration, and in general does not require any laboratory monitoring. ORT avoids the risks of intravenous lines, and the required ingredients are widely available.

When treating dehydration, give 50–100 mL/kg of ORT over the first four hours, depending on the degree of dehydration. Afterwards, reassess the patient and determine whether further care is needed, or if the patient can continue therapy at home. In addition to ORT, encourage breastfeeding when possible, and provide foods such as the BRAT diet (bananas, rice, applesauce, toast/starches). Contraindications to ORT include shock, age less than 1 month, severe respiratory distress, severely altered sensorium, painful abdominal distension, and bowel ileus (check for bowel sounds prior to providing ORT).

Traditionally, ORT solutions have been made with pre-packaged mixtures, or according to the following recipe:

- 3.5 g NaCl (providing 90 mEq/L of Na+)

- 1.5 g KCl (providing 20 mEq/L of K+)

- 2.5 g sodium bicarbonate (providing 30 mmol/L of HCO_3^-) or 2.9 g trisodium citrate dehydrate

- 20 g glucose (providing 111 mmol/L of dextrose)

- 1 liter clean drinking water

However, recent studies have shown that lowering the osmolarity of the ORT solution to 245 mOsm/L can help decrease stool output and vomiting in most cases. When ORT packets are not available, local supplies can be used to create such a solution. One basic recipe:

Cook 100 grams of rice in 1 liter clean drinking water for 10 minutes. Drain all of the water from the rice into a container (try to squeeze out as much water as possible from the rice). Then add a pinch of salt, and enough water to bring the total volume to 1 liter. Carrot soup or rice carrot soup are old Asian remedies for treatment of children with diarrhea. These are well tolerated and effective.

Caring for the Child Health Provider

When working with children who have diarrhea, it is crucial that caretakers wash hands frequently and avoid getting instruments contaminated with stool. Shigella has been cultured for as long as 17 days after inoculation on a toilet seat or medical instrument. If hand-washing facilities are not available, carry Purell or another alcohol-based lotion for hand disinfection.

Sources

"Infant Nutrition During a Disaster: Breastfeeding and Other Options." AAP, 2007. Available at: http://www2.aap.org/breastfeeding/files/pdf/InfantNutritionDisaster.pdf

"Infant Feeding in Emergencies." Emergency Nutrition Network, 2007. Available at: http://www.ennonline.net/pool/files/ife/module-2-v1-1-complete-english.pdf

"Traditional Medicine (Fact Sheet No. 134)". WHO (World Health Organization), 2008. Available at: http://www.who.int/mediacentre/factsheets/fs134/en/index.html

Debas HT, Laxminarayan R, Straus SE. "Complementary and Alternative Medicine". In: Jamison DT, Breman JG, Measham AR, et al., editors. Disease Control Priorities in Developing Countries. 2nd edition. Washington (DC): World Bank; 2006. Chapter 69. Available from: http://www.ncbi.nlm.nih.gov/books/NBK11796/

Oshikoya KA, Sammons HM, Choonara I. A systematic review of pharmacokinetics studies in children with protein-energy malnutrition. Eur J Clin Pharmacol (2010) 66:1025–1035.

Gura KM, Chan LN. 2008. Drug Therapy and Role of Nutrition. In: Duggan C, et al. Nutrition in Pediatrics. 4th ed. Hamilton, Ontario, Canada: BC Decker Inc. 191–208.

"Gate Theory." Buzzy Personal Pain Control. MMJ Labs. June 9, 2013. Available at: http://www.buzzy4shots.com/Hospital/gate-theory.html

"Emergency Triage Assessment and Treatment (ETAT): Manual for participants." WHO. 2005. Available at: http://whqlibdoc.who.int/publications/2005/9241546875_eng.pdf

"Integrated Management of Childhood Illness." WHO. 2008. Available at: http://whqlibdoc.who.int/publications/2008/9789241597289_eng.pdf

Pediatric Hospital Medicine Manual. WHO.2010.

"Enterohaemorrhagic Escherichia coli (EHEC): Fact Sheet No. 125". WHO (World Health Organization), 2011. Available at: http://www.who.int/mediacentre/factsheets/fs125/en/

23. Obstetrics and Newborn Resuscitation

Dr. Denise Lopez Domowicz

PLANNING AND PREPARATION

Establishing appropriate policies and care paths for pregnant women and newborns in complex humanitarian emergencies (CHEs) can prevent a significant amount of morbidity and mortality. In all CHE situations, pregnant women, post-partum women and newborns must be identified as vulnerable populations. These women and infants should receive priority access to medical care, transportation and secure rations. Policies should be established to promote breast-feeding; lactating women should receive additional rations due to their increased caloric needs. Once in the late or recovery phase of a CHE, all women of childbearing age should receive a tetanus booster to prevent neonatal tetanus.

Health care workers should become aware of local resources, birthing customs and cultural practices of newborn care. In many cases, the local population will be able to provide additional birthing resources. These resources may be best identified with the help of community leaders. Health care workers should identify local hospital and clinics, midwives, traditional healers and traditional birth attendants. All of these elements can be incorporated into birthing algorithms.

Birthing algorithms should be prepared in advance, so that they are available as a guide at the time of labor. The majority of births can be successfully completed in the field with minimal intervention from health care workers. Health care workers should be able to identify high-risk births, realize the capabilities of the field hospital, realize the capabilities of referral hospitals and have a safe, reliable method of transportation identified in advance.

DANGER SIGNS IN PREGNANCY

All pregnant women should be monitored for complications. The following list can serve as a screening tool to identify women who need more careful evaluation and possible intervention:

- Headaches.
- Vaginal bleeding.
- Fever.
- Swelling of face or hands.
- Blurred vision.
- Abdominal pain.
- Severe anemia/malaria.
- Multiple pregnancy.
- Prior stillbirth or neonatal death.

PREPARATIONS FOR BIRTH

Health care workers should make certain that all of the basic equipment for newborn delivery and resuscitation are assembled and, above all, CLEAN prior to delivery. The following is an example of a basic equipment list:

- Two pieces of string (each roughly one foot long).
- A razor blade or sharp scissors.
- A bar of soap.
- Four pieces of cloth (one to wash the infant's eyes, one to wipe the infant, one to wash the mother's genitals after birth, one to clean up after the birth).
- A bulb suction.
- Neonatal face mask.
- Neonatal Ambu bag.
- Gentian violet.

138

- Laryngoscope and endotracheal tube for removal of meconium.
- Gloves.

The most important aspect of all births is to maintain cleanliness. The razor blade and the strings must be boiled and cooled. The strings should be left in the water until used. Health care workers should wash their hands and forearms with soap and water, wash the mother's genitals and wash their hands again. When available, gloves should be worn and universal precautions followed to protect the infant, mother and health care worker.

STAGES OF LABOR

First Stage of Labor

During the first stage of labor, the muscles of the uterus tighten and relax in order to push the baby down and out, causing the cervix (the opening of the uterus) to open. During this stage, the mother experiences increasing pain in her lower abdomen and back. Bloody mucous and/or a gush of blood from the vagina is normal. The pains come at regular times and are accompanied by hardening of the abdomen. The mother should rest between the pains. **Vaginal exams are not necessary; they increase the risk of infection and may cause discomfort to the mother.**

During the first stage of labor, the involvement of a traditional birth attendant can be priceless. To help during this stage, the health care worker can:

- Suggest that the mother frequently change position to be more comfortable (walking, squatting, moving from side to side, using hands to pull knees up).

- Talk to the mother and reassure her that everything is okay.

- Make sure that the equipment is ready to go.

- Make sure mother passes urine frequently (a full bladder can obstruct delivery of the baby or cause postpartum hemorrhage).

Danger signs in labor

- Hemorrhage.
- Cord prolapse.
- Abnormal presentation (breech, brow, arm, shoulder).
- Shoulder dystocia.

Second Stage of Labor

The second stage of labor is when the baby passes down the birth canal and out the vagina. During this stage, pains will come every two minutes or less. **Do not leave the patient** when the pains are strong and coming often. Rectal pressure increases similar to the pressure of a bowel movement. The mother wants to push. Coach the mother to push when she feel pain and rest when the pain stops. When the mother has pushed several times, the head of the baby will stay in the opening.

Put your hand on the baby's head to stop it from coming out too quickly. In most cases, the baby's head will be face down during delivery. Put your hand against the part of the mother where the baby's face will come (below the vagina) to support the tissues and support the descent of the head. Take the baby's head in both hands and **lower it down very carefully** to help the top shoulder come out first. Then raise the head to ease the bottom shoulder up and out. If the shoulders do not come out easily, first call for help and then open mother's legs as wide as possible. Try and rotate, or corkscrew, the infant by sliding your hands along the shoulders (not the head). If this fails, you may have to cut an episiotomy, which is a small, midline incision of the mother's tissue from the posterior vaginal opening towards the rectum. If the above steps fail, you may have to reach in and try to deliver the posterior arm. Put your hand on the bottom shoulder blade and "sweep" the arm across the baby's chest. **NEVER, NEVER, NEVER PULL ON THE BABY'S HEAD!!!**

Using the boiled strings, tie the umbilical cord in two places close to the infant, about an inch apart. Using the boiled razor or scissors, cut the cord between the two knots. Protect your eyes, since blood may spurt from the umbilical cord when cut.

Third Stage of Labor

The third stage of labor involves the delivery of the placenta. The placenta should come out easily. Never pull on the cord. Delivery of the placenta can be slow and may take up to an hour. When the placenta is delivered, it must be examined to see if it is complete. If the placenta does not come out in an hour or if it looks torn with missing pieces, this is not normal; transport to the hospital is the best option.

Some bleeding after delivery of the infant is normal, usually about two to three cups. It is useful for health care workers to practice estimating bleeding by spilling water onto cloths. **It is not normal for the mother to lose more blood after the placenta is out.** Health care providers can try to stop the bleeding through a number of methods:

- Massage the top of the uterus.

- Put the baby to the breast (sucking induces maternal oxytocin).

- Pitocin – 10 mg IM (may be repeated up to 3 times).

- If available, follow with Methergine – 0.2 mg IM.

- Consider intravenous fluids.

- Plan for rapid transport to a hospital, if available.

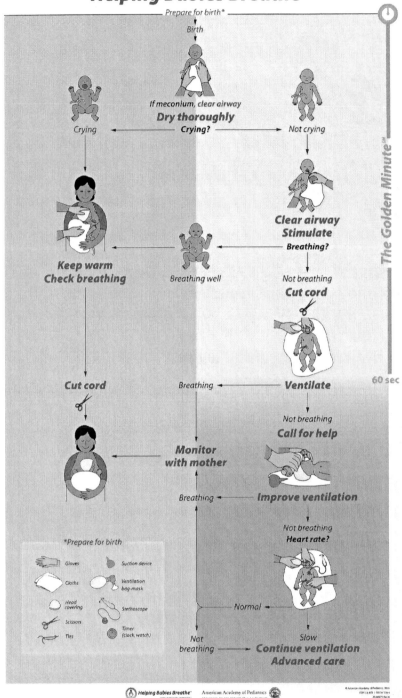

ACTION PLAN
Helping Babies Breathe

Used with permission of the **American Academy of Pediatrics** © 2010, *Helping Babies Breathe Learner Workbook*, ISBN 13: 978–1–58110–354–0, www.helpingbabiesbreathe.org,

24. Care of the Neonate

Neonates are a vulnerable population who need special attention. There is growing evidence that the presence of a well-prepared and skilled health care provider at birth improves neonatal outcome. This chapter covers: 1) Basic resuscitation principles, shown to improve neonatal death and give a better start to babies who struggle to breathe at birth. 2) Principal measures to prevent, recognize and treat neonatal infection in a resource limited setting. 3) Evaluation and management of hyperbilirubinemia in newborns.

BASIC PRINCIPLES DURING DELIVERY

Along with many partners, the American Academy of Pediatrics initiated the Helping Babies Breathe (HBB) program, a neonatal resuscitation curriculum for resource limited settings. Helping Babies Breathe emphasizes the presence of skilled birth attendants, assessment of every baby, temperature support, stimulation to breathe, and assisted ventilation as needed, all within "The Golden Minute"© after birth. Please refer to the information on the Helping Babies Breathe graphic reprinted here with written permission from the Academy of Pediatrics.

Neonates have immature immune systems and are at increased risk for infection. The following aseptic care principles are essential during delivery:

- Clean hands with proper hand washing and sanitizing
- Clean sheets for drying and swaddling
- Clean blade to cut the cord and a clean umbilical cord tie.

Neonates are also at risk for temperature instability. The following measures to prevent hypothermia should be taken. Provide a warm birth environment. Dry the newborn with clean towels. Hand the newborn to mother for Kangaroo care (skin-to-skin contact). Postpone bathing as it is not necessary in the first day of life. If transport to another facility is needed, use a thermal wrap to decrease the risk of hypothermia. In the case of premature labor, efforts should be done to transfer the mother to a health care facility; especially if less than 32 weeks gestation.

A crying newborn who is vigorous and has good tone does not need intervention. The newborn should be dried with a clean towel and handed directly to the mother before clamping the cord. Suctioning the mouth and nose is not required in spontaneously breathing babies born through clear amniotic fluid.

Delaying cord clamping to after 1 minute of life improves neonatal outcome. Clamping the umbilical cord should be performed after 1 minute of life but no later than 3 minutes of life. The use of a timer clock allows for clamping the cord at the ideal time. Using the boiled strings, tie the umbilical cord in two places close to the infant, about an inch apart. Using the boiled razor or scissors, cut the cord between the two knots. Protect your eyes, since blood may spurt from the umbilical cord when cut.

The apneic baby

Approximately ten percent of babies are born limp or with poor or no respiratory effort requiring intervention. If the newborn is not crying or is limp, start by drying with a clean towel; then stimulate by gently rubbing the back 2–3 times and clear the airway using bulb suction. If crying or breathing starts during or after these basic measures, place the newborn on the mother's chest and cut the cord (after 1 minute). If the baby remains limp or not breathing, cut the cord then transfer the newborn to a clean surface and initiate positive pressure ventilation.

Positive pressure ventilation should be started within one minute if the newborn remains apneic after drying and stimulation. A self-inflating bag and face mask interface is the preferred modality and is used in most settings to provide positive pressure breaths. Bag and mask ventilation (BMV) is a skill that improves with training. Maintain a good seal and monitor chest rise during ventilation. If chest rise is inadequate, suction the nasopharynx (mouth and nose); then gently resume BMV keeping the rate at 40 breaths per minute. Adequate BMV is assessed by both good chest rise and monitoring heart rate every 60 seconds.

Monitor the heart rate by using a stethoscope or palpating the umbilical cord. The heart rate should remain at more than 100 beats per minute. If the heart rate is less that 100 beats per minute, make sure appropriate ventilation is performed. The heart rate improves with appropriate ventilation in the vast majority of cases. In newborns more than 32 weeks gestational age, ventilation is performed with room air. The vast majority of newborns start crying or breathing after only few positive pressure breaths. Call for help if the newborn does not start breathing or crying with BMV.

Meconium stained amniotic fluid

Meconium in the amniotic fluid (meconium stained) requires special attention only if the newborn is not crying or breathing spontaneously. Suctioning the nasopharynx is not needed if the newborn is vigorous and routine newborn care is initiated as described above. If the newborn is not breathing or limp, tracheal suction should be performed only if a skilled birth attendant is available; otherwise suction the mouth and nose gently before starting positive pressure ventilation.

When to stop

The World Health Organization (WHO) 2012 guidelines recommend that resuscitation efforts are stopped after 10 minutes if no spontaneous heart rate is documented. If the heart rate was persistently less than 60 beats per minute intervention may be stopped at 20 minutes of life.

146

25.   Neonatal Sepsis

The risk of neonatal infection in resource limited settings may be higher due to unsafe birthing practices. Prevention, early recognition and appropriate treatment of neonatal infection are crucial.

Key risk factors for neonatal infection include: maternal fever ≥ 38°C, chorioamnioitis, prolonged rupture of membranes (> 18–24 hours), foul smelling amniotic fluid, preterm labor, urinary tract infection, group B streptococcus (GBS) colonization, history of a sibling with sepsis, prematurity, low birth weight, low Apgar scores (≤ 6 at 5 minutes of life).

Sick newborns present with non-specific signs and symptoms. Clinical findings may be subtle such as difficulty feeding, excessive sleepiness, irritability, or more noticeable such as fever, respiratory distress (grunting, chest wall retractions), apnea (cessation of breathing for more than 15–20 seconds), tachypnea (respiratory rate > 60 breath per minute), cyanosis, convulsions, bulging fontanel, or abdominal distention. The umbilical cord area should be left without a dressing and checked for signs of infection (discharge/pus draining, surrounding skin redness, swelling or tenderness).

Point-of-care testing, when combined with current algorithms and clinical judgment, may improve our clinical diagnostic abilities. Even though point-of-care testing technology has been available for a long time, operational challenges continue to exist in low-income countries (supply chain, personnel training, equipment maintenance, and quality assurance). In addition, there are no current recommendations or guidance from the WHO and other normative bodies in regards to risk-benefit and cost-effectiveness of point-of-care testing. However, within a few years point-of-care testing may be available to improve our ability to diagnose sick newborns in resource poor areas.

Etiology

The etiology of neonatal sepsis is continually evolving and varies by age and location. Early onset sepsis is defined as infection in the first week of life. It is thought to be transmitted prenatally or during delivery. Late onset sepsis occurs after the first week of life and is usually acquired after birth. Gram negative bacteria (E. Coli, Klebsiella Spp. and Pseudomonas, Acinetobacter, others) account for two thirds of neonatal sepsis. Gram positive cocci (staphylococcus aureus, group B streptococcus, others) cause the other third.

Treatment

In 2002 the WHO published simplified anti-microbial regimens for treatment of neonatal sepsis and later added these to the Pocket Book for the Hospital Care in Children. Recent evidence raises concerns regarding the efficacy of these regimens. Empiric antibiotic therapy should take into consideration local prevalence and anti-microbial susceptibility. Figure 1 summarizes antibiotic options for the facility setting, pending new evidence-based comprehensive recommendations for neonatal infection treatment. In the community, gentamicin intramuscular (IM) in combination with either amoxicillin 15 mg/kg/dose orally every 12 hours or procaine benzylpenicillin 50,000 units/kg/dose IM every 24 hours. Cefuroxime 50 mg/kg/dose PO (1st week of life: every 12 hrs; 2nd – 4th week of life: every 8 hrs) is a reasonable alternative. Transfer the neonate immediately to a health care facility if there is worsening in clinical status or no improvement in 24 to 48 hours after initiation of therapy.

Neonatal Sepsis Diagram

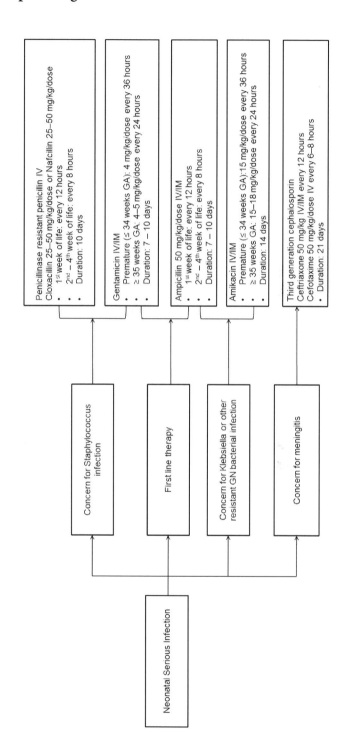

Empiric antibiotic therapy for the facility setting. Ampicillin and gentamicin are suitable first line therapy. If Staphylococcus infection is suspected (example: abscess, excessive skin pustules) or bone/joint infection or omphalitis (umbilical cord infection), replace Ampicillin with a penicillinase resistant penicillins. If no improvement is noted and gram negative (GN) bacterial infection is suspected, replace gentamicin with Amikacin. If meningitis is suspected, add a third generation cephalosporin (Ceftriaxone, Cefotaxime) for better cerebrospinal fluid penetration. Intravenous (IV), intramuscular (IM).

26. Hyperbilirubinemia

Kernicterus due to newborn hyperbilirubinemia continues to be a major cause of death and disability in many countries. Nine per cent of newborn deaths in African hospitals are due to hyperbilirubinemia. Many children survive infancy but with deafness, motor and cognitive impairments. A major cause of hyperbilirubinemia relates to use of inappropriate medications or skin ointments in infants with G6PD deficiency. Around 400 million people are affected worldwide; 10% of Africans and up to 20% of persons of Mediterranean decent have G6PD deficiency. Skin preparations containing naphthalene or mentholatum can lead to hemolysis and hyperbilirubinemia in G6PD deficient infants.

The Bilistik is a practical point-of-care device to measure plasma bilirubin in infants. It requires 25 microliters of blood and provides a measure in 100 seconds. The recorder costs $200 and the testing strip 15 cents.

Light treatment bilirubin levels vary by both gestational age (GA) and postnatal age (PNA). Conservative light treatment bilirubin levels are summarized in table 1. Continue light treatment until bilirubin levels reach 1–2 mg/dl below initiation levels. Start light treatment at lower bilirubin levels in sick newborns. Consult with a specialist and consider exchange transfusion if the bilirubin level is 8–10 mg/dl above light treatment level. The appropriate use of blue light bulbs includes attention to lining the bassinet with white cloth, distance from the bulbs, number of bulbs and age of bulbs. Blue bulbs used for 2,000 hours will no longer provide sufficient radiance for phototherapy.

Selectively filtered sunlight phototherapy is effective and safe if used appropriately. Tents with specific film covers for cloudy and sunny days have been devised to provide mainly blue transmitted light. Infants must be checked often for temperature and sunburn.

Table - Light Treatment

Light Treatment Level Based on Gestational Age (GA) and Postnatal Age (PNA)				
	Term	Late Preterm	Preterm	
PNA	GA > 37 wks	GA 35 – 37 wks	GA 33 – 34 wks	GA ≤ 32 wks
0–24 hrs	Any Visible Jaundice	Any Visible Jaundice	6 mg/dl	5 mg/dl
25–36 hrs	10 mg/dl	8 mg/dl	8 mg/dl	5 mg/dl
37–48 hrs	12 mg/dl	10 mg/dl	8 mg/dl	6 mg/dl
49–72 hrs	15 mg/dl	12 mg/dl	10 mg/dl	8 mg/dl
> 72 hrs	18 mg/dl	15 mg/dl	12 mg/dl	10 mg/dl

Recommended Readings and References

Helping Babies Breathe; http://www.helpingbabiesbreathe.org

World Health Organization, Guidelines on basic newborn resuscitation, 2012.

World Health Organization, Explore simplified antimicrobial regimens for the treatment of neonatal sepsis. Geneva, 30th September – 1st October 2002.

Jani I, Trevor P. How Point-of-Care Testing Could Drive Innovation in Global Health. NEJM, June 2013.

27. Biochemical Terrorism

Dr. Jordana Hikri

Biochemical terrorism refers to the use of biological, chemical, or radioactive agents against a civilian population. Biochemical terrorism has been around for thousands of years. In the sixth century BCE, the Assyrians used rye ergot to poison the wells of their enemies. During the Tartars' siege of Kaffa (modern-day Feodosiya, Ukraine) in the mid-fourteenth century, plague-ridden bodies of dead soldiers were flung over the city's walls in order to infect the besieged population. World War II saw the use of chemical agents against the Nazis victims, as well as much research into biological terrorism by both the Japanese and the Allied Forces. Certainly, biochemical terrorism has continued into the 21st century, as evidenced by the anthrax-laden letters delivered in the aftermath of September 11th, 2001. More recently, the alleged use of chemical weapons in Syria's civil war has renewed talk of biochemical terrorism.

Special Issues for Children in Biochemical terrorism

Children's unique physiology can increase their odds of a negative outcome when faced with biochemical terrorism. A child's shorter stature, combined with the tendency of many chemical and nuclear agents to settle close to the ground, increases the child's exposure to these agents. Children's higher respiratory rate and minute volume increases their exposure to inhaled infectious and chemical agents. Children's higher surface-to-volume ratio makes them more prone to absorbable toxins. In addition, younger children, and those with physical or intellectual disabilities, are less able to physically remove themselves from harm's way, or to anticipate danger.

Even if children are not physically injured by a biochemical attack, they may have serious psychological injuries. Parents, teachers, neighbors or playmates may be severely injured or may die. Homes and neighborhoods may be destroyed or made uninhabitable. Children may be displaced to unfamiliar environments. They may be frightened by television or radio coverage of the attack. All of this may lead to acute anxiety and depression, as well as to long-term psychological issues.

Responding to Biochemical Terrorism

The first step in responding to biochemical terrorism is to be prepared. Have a plan, conduct drills, and know how to initiate the emergency chain of response. Know the signs and symptoms of various toxic exposures, keeping in mind that exposures may be multifactorial—for example, a "dirty bomb" may cause both conventional blast injuries, as well as radiation sickness.

When a biochemical attack happens, the primary goal must be maintaining the safety of first responders and unaffected civilians, while saving as many lives as possible. To this end, the incident commander should set up various response zones. The "hot zone" is where the attack directly struck. The hot zone may contain non-neutralized threats, and as such it should be marked off, with entry forbidden to all but the most necessary personnel. Ideally, patients should not be treated in the hot zone (beyond the initial Airway-Breathing-Circulation of CPR), but should be moved to an adjacent "warm zone", where they can be decontaminated if needed, and stabilized for transport. To aid in decontamination, the warm zone" should preferably be upwind or uphill from the hot zone. Finally, patients can be moved to the "cool," or "support," zone, for ongoing care. It is to everyone's advantage to keep media and other non-essential personnel out of all of the response zones.

Keep in mind the upside-down triage triangle: ▽ This symbol serves to remind us that in general, the least sick (the "walking wounded" and the "worried well") will be the first to arrive to the hospital. Those that are closest to the hot zone, trapped, or severely injured, however, will arrive later—and in smaller numbers.

Some Specific Biologic and Chemical Agents

While some terrorist attacks may be blatant, others may have very subtle presentations, or concealed secondary elements. The initial signs and symptoms of various biochemical agents may mimic naturally-occurring illnesses. Even when one cannot identify the causal agent, however, remember that seemingly minor details—such as the chronology of a rash, or the odor associated with a chemical exposure—may be crucial in identifying the etiology.

What follows is a brief review of some of the most significant biochemical terrorism agents, written with the intention of providing an introduction to their presentations and treatments. A great deal of additional information is available on the CDC and AAP websites.

Biological Agents

The CDC classifies biological agents based on their transmissibility, mortality, and potential for weaponization. The following are those agents listed under Category A—the highest risk category.

Anthrax (Bacillus anthracis):

There are three forms of anthrax: cutaneous (contracted via direct contact with spores), inhalation, and gastrointestinal (the rarest form, contracted by ingesting contaminated meat or spores). Anthrax is not spread by people. There is currently no anthrax vaccination available for patients under 18 years, but there is a recommended post-exposure prophylactic regimen for children (either ciprofloxacin or doxycycline). The following describes anthrax presentations in children over 2 months of age and adults (the presentations in infants under 2 months of age is not well described in the literature).

Cutaneous anthrax has an incubation period of 1–12 days, and progresses from a painless papule to a vesicular lesion, finally forming a central black eschar. The lesion may be associated with fever, headache, and regional lymphadenopathy. Although the mortality rate is 20%, this falls to <1% when appropriate antibiotic therapy (ciprofloxacin or doxycycline) is given.

Inhalation anthrax has an incubation period of 1–7 days, though occasionally the period can be as long as 60 days. The disease begins with a brief prodrome of influenza-like respiratory symptoms, progressing to dyspnea and shock, with radiographic evidence of mediastinal widening and pleural effusion. Patients often develop meningitis as well. Inhalation anthrax has a very high mortality rate, despite appropriate multi-drug treatment regimens.

Gastrointestinal anthrax has an incubation period of 1–7 days, and is characterized by severe abdominal pain followed by fever and signs of septicemia. There may also be oral lesions, dysphagia, nausea, and hematemesis or bloody diarrhea. It is not clear whether antibiotics affect the mortality rate, which is estimated at 25% – 60%. Gastrointestinal anthrax is treated identically to pulmonary anthrax.

Botulism (Clostridium botulinum toxin):

Unlike naturally-occurring forms of botulism (e.g. foodborne or wound botulism), inhalational botulism does not occur naturally— rather, it is the result of the release of aerosolized botulism toxin. Unfortunately, it cannot be distinguished clinically from naturally-occurring forms of botulism. Keep in mind that the incubation period for foodborne botulism (6 hours – 10 days) may be shorter with inhaled toxin. Symptoms include symmetric descending weakness and flaccid paralysis, along with cranial neuropathies. Patients are generally afebrile, with normal sensation and mentation. Treatment is supportive (and may include ventilatory support), though antitoxin may prevent or decrease symptoms.

Plague (Yersinia pestis)

Naturally harbored in the fleas of certain rodents, aerosolized plague bacteria could (after a 1–6 day incubation period) cause pneumonic plague. While bubonic plague is generally spread via flea bites, pneumonic plague can be spread from person to person via respiratory droplets. Symptoms include fever and rapidly developing pneumonia, sometimes with hemoptysis. The buboes of the eponymous bubonic plague are not seen in primary pneumonic plague (although untreated cases of bubonic plague can progress to the pneumonic form). Untreated, pneumonic plague can rapidly lead to respiratory failure and shock. Available antibiotics used in the treatment of plague include tetracyclines, fluoroquinolones, streptomycin, and gentamicin.

Smallpox (variola major):

Although naturally-occurring smallpox has been eliminated around the world, there remains the potential for the deliberate release of (likely aerosolized) variola virus. The resultant disease has a roughly 30% mortality rate. Generally spread via respiratory droplets, body fluids, or contaminated household items (e.g. linen), infection is followed by a 7–17 (on average 12) day incubation period, during which the patient is asymptomatic and non-contagious. This is followed by a 2–4 day prodrome of high fever and severe malaise, during which the patient may be contagious. A raised, spotted rash then appears—first in the mouth, then on the face, rapidly spreading outward to the extremities. As soon as the rash appears, the patient is certainly contagious. The rash slowly transforms into firm round pustules, which after roughly five days will begin to scab over. Roughly three weeks after the first appearance of the rash, all of the scabs will have fallen off, and the patient will no longer be contagious.

Keep in mind that smallpox could potentially be confused for chickenpox (varicella). The two rashes, however, differ in several ways. Whereas smallpox lesions are deep and appear simultaneously, varicella lesions are more superficial and come in crops, allowing the clinician to appreciate lesions in varying stages of maturity. In addition, the lesions of smallpox tend to be concentrated on the face and limbs, whereas chickenpox are found more on the trunk. Finally, although varicella is now a recommended routine vaccination, people are no longer vaccinated against smallpox. In the event of a smallpox outbreak, the only method of treatment is vaccination, either given prophylactically or within three days of exposure. Significant contraindications exist to smallpox vaccination, however, including a personal history of, or household member with, any of the following: atopic dermatitis, immunodeficiency, pregnancy, and age under 12 months. All contraindications must be weighed carefully in the face of a true smallpox emergency.

Tularemia (Francisella tularensis)

Naturally found in rodents and rabbits, Francisella tularensis is an extremely infective bacterium that is most commonly spread via the bite of infected insects, or by handling infected animals. Less often, tularemia is spread via contaminated food or water, or via inhalation. Tularemia is not known to employ person-to-person transmission. Following a 1–14 (on average 3–5) day incubation period, symptoms emerge. Cutaneous contact can cause ulcers and painful lymphadenopathy. Inhalation (e.g. following an aerosolized release) can lead to the abrupt onset of fever, flu-like symptoms, pneumonia, hemoptysis, and respiratory failure. Tularemia can be fatal without appropriate treatment, which includes tetracyclines, fluoroquinolones, streptomycin, or gentamicin.

Viral hemorrhagic fevers

Viral hemorrhagic fevers (VHF) are caused by at least four viral families: arenaviruses (including Lassa and Machupo), filoviruses (including Ebola and Marburg), bunyaviruses, and flaviviruses. The viruses that cause VHF are not naturally hosted by humans. In some cases, however, infected humans can transmit the infection to others. Symptoms vary by specific virus, but in general include high fever and malaise. More serious cases involve cutaneous, internal, or mucosal bleeding, although patients rarely die from VHF-associated bleeding. The most serious cases of VHF develop shock, nervous system dysfunction, and/or renal failure. With few exceptions, VHFs have no specific preventative or therapeutic agents. Treatment, therefore, is focused on supportive care, and the prevention of new infections by controlling zoonotic vectors and isolating infected individuals.

Nerve Agents

Nerve agents such as GA (tabun), GB (sarin), GD (soman), and VX, are among the most toxic chemical agents that have been used in biochemical terrorist attacks. Originally intended as pesticides, these difficult-to-detect chemicals were rapidly adopted by militaries and terrorist organizations. Indeed, in 1995 a religious cult released sarin gas on a Tokyo subway, leaving thirteen dead and more than 5,500 injured.

Whether via inhalation, ingestion, or direct skin and mucosal contact, nerve agents can rapidly lead to cholinergic crisis via inhibition of acetylcholinesterase. Symptoms may include rhinorrhea, salivation, sweating, pinpoint pupils, shortness of breath, chest tightness, nausea, vomiting, involuntary evacuation, seizures, paralysis, coma, and respiratory failure. Death can occur within 1–10 minutes. Conversely, the effect of more modest dermal exposure may be delayed for up to 18 hours. If one survives the initial exposure, neurological complications (such as irritability, fatigue, and memory deficits) may persist for months.

After removing the patient from the hot zone and performing decontamination, the antidotes atropine and pralidoxime chloride (2–PAM Cl) should be administered intramuscularly, per the recommended age-appropriate dosing: 0.05–0.1 mg/kg of atropine (maximum 2–4 mg/dose), and 15–25 mg/kg 2–PAM Cl. If symptoms persist, give an additional dose of atropine every 5–10 minutes until respiratory symptoms subside. If the military Mark I antidote autoinjector kits are available, know that one autoinjector contains 2 mg atropine and the other 600 mg of 2–PAM Cl — potentially a larger-than-anticipated dose in a pediatric patient.

RADIATION

Whether as the result of an accident (such as the 2011 Fukushima nuclear disaster in Japan) or an act of terrorism, children who are exposed to harmful radiation are especially at risk for negative effects (as discussed earlier in this chapter). Following decontamination, children should be admitted to a hospital for monitoring and treatment. Anyone exposed to radiation should have their individual dose assessment calculated. This assessment is based on a number of clinical and laboratory values, such as the timing of the onset of nausea/vomiting, the trajectory of lymphopenia on serial CBCs, and the presence of peripheral chromosomal abnormalities. The assessment of total body radiation is made in grays (Gy), where 1 Gy = 100 rads.

Treatment for radiation exposure depends on the type of radiation encountered, as well as the severity of exposure. Radioiodines, for example, are often released following nuclear power plant disasters. These isotopes are known to target the thyroid, thereby increasing the lifetime risk of thyroid cancer. Any child exposed to greater than 0.05 Gy of radioiodine should therefore be treated with potassium iodide (KI). When given prior to (or as soon as possible following) exposure, KI can help prevent radioiodine uptake. If required, additional doses should be given every 24 hours. Keep in mind that even once the initial exposure has ceased, potential sources of ongoing exposure include breast milk, animal milk, and local produce. Therefore, these items should be avoided as much as possible, until deemed safe by public health authorities. Once all radioiodine exposure has ceased, infants will still require ongoing monitoring of thyroid function tests.

KI has only mild side effects including rash and gastrointestinal upset. KI is available in 65 mg and 130 mg tablets. Dosing is based on age, and a solution can be prepared for younger children as follows:

Guidelines for Preparation of KI Solution Using the 65 mg tablet:

- Put one 65 mg KI tablet into a small bowl and grind into a fine powder. Do not leave any large pieces.

- Add 20 mL of water to the KI powder and mix until dissolved.

- Add 20 mL of juice, soda, or syrup (to help disguise the taste) to the KI/water mixture and mix well.

- The resulting mixture has 8.125 mg of KI per 5 mL, and will keep for seven days if refrigerated.

Age-based dosing guidelines for KI:

- Newborn through one month of age = 16 mg (roughly 10 mL)

- One month through three years of age = 32 mg (roughly 20 mL)

- Four years through 17 years of age = 65 mg (roughly 40 mL, or one 65-mg tablet)

- Greater than 17 years of age or weight greater than 70 kg = 130 mg (two 65-mg tablets)

Helping Children Cope

Adults caring for children in the aftermath of biochemical terrorism must be aware of their own psychological state, as children are much better at "reading" adults than one may appreciate. Talk with the child about what has happened, and try to understand his or her view of the situation. Encourage the child to ask questions. Caretakers should attempt to reestablish daily routines as soon as possible. Remember that the child's psychological response to biochemical terrorism may vary, depending on the age, past experiences, and developmental stage. Keep in mind that fear and anxiety, even if initially hidden, may manifest in multiple ways for months or even years to come. See the chapter on Development and Mental Health for more guidance on these issues.

"History of Biological Warfare." NPR. Oct. 18, 2001. Available online at: http://www.npr.org/news/specials/response/anthrax/features/2001/oct/011018.bioterrorism.history.html

Lehman-Huskamp KL, Keenan WJ, Scalzo AJ, Yin S. "Toxic Exposures." In Pediatric Education in Disasters. AAP, 2008: 5–

Wathen J, Cooper L, Crossman K, Acosta Bastidas M. "Pediatric Trauma." In Pediatric Education in Disasters. AAP, 2008: 28.

"Children and Anthrax: A Fact Sheet for Clinicians." CDC. Nov. 8, 2001. Available online at: http://www.bt.cdc.gov/agent/anthrax/pediatricfactsheet.asp

"Botulism Facts for Health Care Providers." CDC. April 19, 2006. Available online at: http://www.bt.cdc.gov/agent/botulism/hcpfacts.asp

"Frequently Asked Questions About Plague." CDC. April 5, 2005. Available online at: http://www.bt.cdc.gov/agent/plague/faq.asp

"Smallpox Disease Overview." CDC. Feb. 6, 2007. Available online at: http://www.bt.cdc.gov/agent/smallpox/overview/disease-facts.asp

"What You Should Know About a Smallpox Outbreak." CDC. Mar. 13, 2009. Available online at: http://www.bt.cdc.gov/agent/smallpox/basics/outbreak.asp

Smallpox (Vaccinia) Vaccine Contraindications. CDC. Feb. 7, 2007. Available online at: http://www.bt.cdc.gov/agent/smallpox/vaccination/contraindications-clinic.asp

"Frequently Asked Questions About Tularemia." CDC. Oct. 8, 2003. Available online at: http://www.bt.cdc.gov/agent/tularemia/faq.asp

"Viral Hemorrhagic Fevers." CDC. June 19, 2013. Available online at: http://www.cdc.gov/ncidod/dvrd/spb/mnpages/dispages/vhf.htm

"Medical Management Guidelines for Nerve Agents: Tabun (GA); Sarin (GB); Soman (GD); and VX." Agency for Toxic Substances and Disease Registry. March 3, 2011. Available online at: http://www.atsdr.cdc.gov/MMG/MMG.asp?id=523&tid=93#bookmark03

Locker, M. "Tokyo Sarin Gas Attack Suspect Arrested, 17 Years Later." Time. June 4, 2012.

28.   Landmines

The landmine crisis is well recognized as a global catastrophe. Although determining exact statistics from individual regions is difficult, the following estimates from the International Committee of the Red Cross (ICRC) illustrate the scope of the problem. Over the past 20 years, hundreds of thousands of people have been killed or maimed by landmines. Each day, landmines kill 30 people and maim countless others. In Cambodia alone, there is an estimated 1 amputee per 236 people. According to United Nations (UN) estimates, it would take 1,100 years to clear the 110 million active landmines that are in place in 64 countries. Prior to the Ottawa convention to ban landmines in 1997, an additional two million mines were being laid annually.

ANTI-PERSONNEL LANDMINES

Anti-personnel landmines were designed to cause more destruction than any other weapon created. They are scattered in areas of combat in order to protect military facilities and restrict enemy movement. Although some mines are designed to result in 100% mortality, many mines are designed to severely injure soldiers. When a soldier is injured by a mine, several people are required to carry, evacuate and care for him. Landmines drain enemy resources and destroy combat morale. Witnessing a land mine injury can cause acute and long-term psychological trauma.

Due to the indiscriminate nature of anti-personnel landmines, civilian populations experience the destructive force of landmines both during and after a conflict. Landmines remain for decades, destroying croplands and devastating communities. Beyond the acute injuries inflicted, landmines diminish future productivity through blindness, deafness and loss of limbs. When a land mine survivor is the head of a family, his entire family suffers financially and emotionally. The psychological trauma caused by landmines is significant for all family members, including the children.

CHILDREN AND LANDMINES

The number of civilian, non-combatant land-mine casualties varies based on region, type of mines and political situation. ICRC database estimates that at least 20 percent of landmine victims are children.

There are many reasons why children in disasters are at particular risk of falling victim to anti-personal landmines. Disasters usually create areas of extreme overpopulation. Children often have no safe places in which to play. In this situation, a poorly marked and desolate landmine field becomes an appealing playground ... a wide open field to run in or the perfect building for hide and seek. Many times, children find the actual mines to be attractive toys. This is particularly true when the mines are designed to look like toys. The unpredictability of detonation contributes to the problem. A group of children may play catch with a mine hundreds of times before it explodes.

In order for health care workers to decrease the risk of landmines to children, fundamental precautions must become ingrained in child behavior. One of the most beautiful, and potentially dangerous, qualities of childhood is the ability to be absorbed in fantasy. When children are playing, they may not remember school lessons. Thus, land mine education must be directed to condition behaviors that children display consistently when they are in areas that contain mines. This can be accomplished by repetition of games that are designed to take advantage of their wonderful imaginations. One approach is to use bright and colorful cartoons of children in unsafe, landmine situations as story telling guides. Children can then tell the teacher and one another about the story in the picture and, hopefully, internalize recognition of areas which are likely to be mine infested. This type of interaction also provides children with outlets to express fears and anger related to their experiences with landmines.

Health care workers should educate themselves on the local existence of landmines and how they are marked. Although no universal marker for mine fields has been developed, most communities develop their own systems for marking these areas. These markers should be incorporated into the teaching games so that children become very familiar with them. Children should learn about other markers that suggest the presence of landmines, such as abandoned or exploded cars in fields or shelled out, empty buildings. Children can rehearse scenarios of what to do once in a mine field.

FIRST AID AND ADVOCACY

Prompt first aid is the most effective step to increase the likelihood of recovery from a mine injury. If applied incorrectly, first-aid measures may lead to medical complications. In areas with known mine fields, health care workers need special training in these measures, including stopping obvious external hemorrhage, appropriate use of intravenous fluids and antibiotics, wound immobilization and pain management. When possible, a referral system should be established well in advance. Once stabilized, patients should be transported to the nearest hospital.

In order for the appropriate resources to be made available, health care workers must serve as advocates for those injured by or in danger from anti-personnel mines. The magnitude of the problem must be identified and made known. Hospitals need to be supported with adequate medical supplies, staff and training; medical systems must be remodeled to include extensive rehabilitation and counseling services; landmine survivors need to be empowered to function in society.

29.   International Law

"All human beings are born free and equal in dignity and rights. They are endowed with reason and conscience and should act towards one another in a spirit of brotherhood."

**The Universal Declaration of Human Rights,
The United Nations, Article 1**

Human rights and humanitarian law play an important role in disasters. Because of the chaos and breakdown inherent in disasters, these rights and laws may be the only remaining guide for human conduct following a disaster. They are followed imperfectly on a global level. Yet, each individual effort to adhere to these principles contributes to the goal of worldwide respect for human rights.

There is an important difference between human rights and humanitarian law. The former is a broad set of principles regarding the inherent dignity and respect due to all mankind in all circumstances. The latter is a series of laws that attempt to protect human rights in the context of armed conflict. More recently, attention has focused on the issue of children in the context of human rights.

HUMAN RIGHTS

The Universal Declaration of Human Rights as affirmed by the United Nations (UN) can be read on the worldwide web at http://www.asociety.com/udhr.html. A few key articles are listed here:

Article 2. "Everyone is entitled to all the rights and freedoms set forth in this declaration, without any distinction of any kind, such as race, color, sex, language, religion, political, or other opinion, national or social origin, property, birth or other status. Furthermore, no distinction shall be made on the basis of the political, jurisdictional or international status of the country or territory to which a person belongs, whether it be independent, trust, non-self-governing or under any other limitation of sovereignty."

Article 5. "No one shall be subjected to torture or to cruel, inhuman or degrading treatment or punishment."

Article 14. "(1) Everyone has the right to seek and to enjoy in other countries asylum from persecution. (2) This right may not be invoked in the case of prosecutions genuinely arising from non-political crimes or from acts contrary to the purposes and principles of the United Nations."

Article 25. "(1) Everyone has the right to a standard of living adequate for the health and well-being of himself and of his family, including food, clothing, housing, and medical care and necessary social services, and the right to security in the event of unemployment, sickness, disability, widowhood, old age, or other lack of livelihood in circumstances beyond his control. (2) Motherhood and childhood are entitled to special care and assistance. All children, whether born in or out of wedlock, shall enjoy the same social protection."

INTERNATIONAL HUMANITARIAN LAW

Better known as the Geneva Conventions, these are actually a series of documents developed over decades for the protection of human rights in the context of armed conflict. They provide detailed rules, which parties to the conflict are bound to follow. These rules attempt to balance human rights with military necessity, the latter being those actions that are necessary to overpower the opponent. They apply specifically to the treatment of wounded and sick members of the armed forces (First and Second Convention), the treatment of prisoners of war (Third Convention) and the protection of civilians in time of war (Fourth Convention, Protocols I and II).

The Geneva Conventions specify that wounded and sick members of the armed forces will be respected and cared for without distinction, particularly with respect nationality; that military ambulances and hospitals and their personnel will be respected and protected; and that a red cross on white background is a sign of immunity. The International Committee of the Red Cross (ICRC) is the neutral and independent agency charged with safeguarding these principles.

These international humanitarian laws apply to medical personnel when their own country is engaged in armed conflict or when their government or relief agencies decide to place them at the disposal of one of the armed parties or the ICRC. Medical personnel may be military or civilian and are defined broadly to include all those participating in activities that support medical purposes. This includes personnel who may not be directly involved in the provision of medical care, but provide support services for those who are (e.g. transportation).

The duties of medical personnel are to give humane treatment to sick and wounded persons; to abstain from all acts of hostility; to carry only light weapons for use in their own defense or the defense of the patients for whom they are responsible; to display the sign of the red cross on their chest and back; and to refrain from committing grave breaches or abuses of international humanitarian law. The principal mission of medical personnel is to assure the protection of human life and health. Medical care is to be provided based on medical necessity and without any distinction other than medical criteria. All medical personnel are to abide by the Geneva Oath, which is:

- To exercise his/her profession with conscience and dignity.

- To treat the health of his/her patient as his/her principal concern.

- To respect secrets entrusted to him/her.

- To abstain from any religious, national, racial, political, or social discrimination in the performance of his/her duty.

- To pay absolute respect to human life.

- Not to use his/her medical knowledge against the laws of humanity, even under threat.

In turn, all medical personnel are accorded respect and protection under the law. They have the right to require authorities to provide means and facilities for the discharge of their duties; to access places where their services are necessary; to visit prisoners of war; and to protect themselves and their patients from reprisals. Medical personnel are explicitly protected from being compelled to act contrary to medical ethics or to give information about the wounded and sick in their care. Medical personnel whose country is not a party to the conflict or who are working for a relief agency or the ICRC are exempt from capture and should be returned expeditiously to their party.

Permanent military medical personnel and civilian medical personnel of a party to the conflict may be detained only if their services are required to tend prisoners of war. They may not be required to do work other than that concerned with their medical duties.

The Geneva Conventions make a distinction between military and civilian persons in time of armed conflict. Civilians are those who do not or no longer take any active part in the hostilities. They are afforded respect and protection under the law. Specifically, they are to be provided special safe zones, which contain no military objectives. Starvation or destruction of their means of survival as a method of warfare is prohibited. Slavery is forbidden. Civilian populations are often displaced in time of conflict. Those who remain in their country but not in their homes are called displaced persons. Those who flee to another country are called refugees. Whether displaced or refugees, children constitute large proportions of these civilian groups.

THE CONVENTION ON THE RIGHTS OF THE CHILD

Most countries in the world have ratified the Convention on the Rights of the Child. The United States has signed it but it has not been ratified by Congress. Established by the UN in 1990, the Convention has a section on armed conflicts: "In accordance with their obligations under International Humanitarian laws in armed conflicts, States Parties should take all feasible measures to ensure protection and care of children who are affected by an armed conflict." (Article 38, pt 4)

PRACTICAL CONSIDERATIONS

In reality, there is poor compliance with international humanitarian law and human rights in most disasters, especially with respect to women and children. Most conflicts are multi-faceted and subject to a confusing blend of political, military, economic, ethnic and social forces. In many of the post cold war conflicts, military groups have targeted civilians, including women and children, and medical institutions such as hospitals. The emblems of the red cross or red crescent no longer assure protection. Since the protections afforded by humanitarian law are not universally known or respected, humanitarian aid workers must maintain a high level of personal caution. There are times when personal security issues conflict with the humanitarian mission. Team decisions regarding the balance between human rights, humanitarian assistance, individual responsibility and safety may be necessary.

30.   Ethical Issues

A Universal Declaration of Human Rights exists. International Humanitarian Law exists. Most countries have ratified the Convention on the Rights of the Child.

And most humans, regardless of culture or ethnic background, would agree that innocent children should not suffer. Yet they do suffer enormously in disasters and antecedent conflicts because of ethical breaches.

CHILD COMBATANTS

One ethical breach that currently occurs on a large scale is the use of children as soldiers and perpetrators of violence. For example, in Sierra Leone, children as young as 8 years of age have been forced to commit atrocities against family and friends, which destroys their moral framework. Without this moral framework, children can become frightening and impulsive combatants. Another notable example is the Lord's Resistance Army (LRA) in Northern Uganda, which has kidnapped young children and forced them to participate in brutal raids of local villages, burning homes and killing people with machetes. Young girls have been enslaved by the LRA and subjected to repeated rape.

It may be hard for humanitarian workers to believe that the playful children they encounter in disaster settings have experienced or participated in violent crimes. Even if such children have been perpetrators of violence, they are victims and require compassion and protection from further harm. Information shared by children regarding atrocities they may have committed must be handled with care and confidentiality. While western nations often detain or incarcerate child offenders, this is not a practical approach in disasters. Local leaders should be called upon to develop a plan for rehabilitation and treatment of child combatants. Every attempt should be made to help these children resume normal development, rebuild moral character and reintegrate into the community.

ADVOCACY

Humanitarian workers must be aware of the interplay that occurs between personal, social, political and medical ethics in disasters. There are many different players in disaster settings, including governments, political factions, organizations, humanitarian workers and victims. The principles and values of these disparate groups vary tremendously. Many may be unaware of international human rights and humanitarian law. What can health workers do to uphold ethical principles for children?

Advocacy is probably the most powerful tool and can be used in the field, as well as in home communities. Providing information to organizations, political leaders, the media and colleagues in child health fields about ethical breaches against children is helpful. The public and persons in power need to know that millions of children have been killed or seriously injured in disasters over the last two decades. In disaster settings, childhood injuries are often treated without access to analgesia, anesthesia or surgical facilities. Tens of millions of children have been made homeless or orphaned, have witnessed or experienced violence and have suffered immeasurable psychological trauma as a result of disasters. It is simply unacceptable to stand by as children suffer in these ways.

The Carnegie Commission and the United Nations (UN) have recommended that a UN force be created specifically to protect children in disaster situations. While this is welcome, at the present time it is the local directors of relief programs who have the greatest ability to uphold basic ethical principles on behalf of children. They can do this by stating the question at each planning meeting: "What is best for children?" Directors can also ensure that staff members know the specifics of international law that relate to children. They can organize meetings with workers on the ethics of food distribution, health care, housing and education. They should recognize when conflicts arise related to ethics and children, and facilitate meetings between the disagreeing parties. Relief workers in the field should inform their directors of ethical breaches that affect children. Whistle blowing on behalf of children is never wrong.

31.   Examples: Good and Bad

A POOR SITUATION

As a result of an earthquake there are 20,000 displaced families and 600 unaccompanied minors (orphans). They are directed to a refugee camp area that has little vegetation and no water supply except from rain. Initially families sleep in the open (it is the rainy season). After two weeks UNICEF sends in tents, but they are desert tents and leak with rain. The unaccompanied minors are placed in a cluster of large tents, divided according to age, ranging from toddlers to teenagers. The majority of the younger orphans are naked, and have diarrhea and respiratory infections. Three weeks after establishment of this refugee area, there are still no latrines and no wells.

Two large tents are organized as a clinic and hospital where expatriate volunteer physicians and nurses are working. There has been no survey to identify health personnel among the displaced persons. Large amounts of intravenous (IV) solutions and antibiotics are brought into the camp, sent by NGO relief agencies. No oral rehydration packets are available. The volunteer medical staff are busy from morning until dark (there is no electricity) treating acutely ill children. In the hospital there are no hand washing facilities or toilets.

Food supplies are air-dropped and distributed to heads of families. Since there is no cooking fuel, initial food supplies are Meals Ready to Eat (MRE) rations. The orphan children are fed MRE rations once a day and are also given high protein biscuits. Drinking water is trucked in and distributed to families in jerry cans. Expatriate volunteers carry jerry cans of water to the orphan area and provide the children with cups of water throughout the day. Because of security problems, the volunteers are not allowed to stay with the orphans at night. There are a few refugee adults who volunteer to help the orphan children at night.

The orphan children appear listless and dejected. Clinical diagnoses of tuberculosis, shigella dysentery, and meningococcal meningitis are made. After four weeks, 100 of the unaccompanied minors (primarily infants and toddlers) have died.

What are the priorities? What can be done to improve the present and future situation for the unaccompanied minors?

A GOOD SITUATION

A disaster has developed as a result of ethnic warfare and 100,000 people have become refugees in another country. Half of them are children under 15 years. Most are in excellent nutritional and physical condition at the time they leave their homes. They travel for only a few days before reaching a refugee camp. International relief agencies have anticipated their movement and have already prepared tents and an address system for housing. Safe water and food is available.

Incoming refugees are identified upon entrance with respect to name, sex and age. Identification bands are placed on wrists of children who are younger than 10 years. Upon entrance, refugees are queried with respect to skills. Those with skills in education, social work and health areas are rapidly involved in prevention programs for the refugee camp. Refugees are provided with preventive information related to the use of available food, latrines, water, childcare, safety, environmental hazards and medications. Special attention is paid to nursing and pregnant women; they are given food supplements and vitamins. Plans for birth are discussed and delivery kits prepared.

Parents are given information about the special needs of their children. Unaccompanied minors are identified and photographed rapidly. Photographs are posted throughout the camp in order to facilitate reunification. In the interim, refugee families are identified who will take care of unaccompanied minors as foster parents. Educators establish temporary schools and playground areas within two weeks of the refugee movement. Camp rules include the requirement for school for children ages 6 years and above. Teachers include programs to counteract the stress and anxiety experienced by the children. Relief agencies provide drawing materials, balls for various games and simple musical instruments that are familiar to the refugees. The UNICEF "Return to Happiness" program is adapted and made available to school age children.

Surveys are done with respect to illnesses and nutritional status of both adults and children. Household members are queried regarding whether they have witnessed violence, experienced personal abuse or been separated from family members. Refeeding programs are initiated immediately for malnourished children. Plans are made to involve adults in some form of work, if it appears that their refugee status will persist beyond a few weeks.

Clinics are organized for children under 5 years of age, involving refugees as much as possible. Arrangements are made for all young children to visit these regularly and for immunizations to be updated. When the time comes for transfer to other camps, relocation to other countries or return to their homelands, refugees are provided with records regarding the health and educational status of their children.

32. Resources

Here we list some print and web resources that may be helpful in disasters. This list is not comprehensive, but rather gives a sample of the resources available.

BOOKS AND MANUALS

Control of Communicable Diseases Manual: Ed. David F. Heymann, American Public Health Association 2008. (19th Edition)

Declaration on Human Rights. The United Nations.

Disabled Village Children: A Guide for Community Health Workers, Rehabilitation Workers and Families, 2nd edition. Werner D. Palo Alto: Hesperian Foundation, 1996.

Essential Nutrition Actions: improving maternal, newborn, infant and young children health and nutrition, WHO, 2012.

Facts for Life. UNICEF/WHO/UNESCO, 4th Edition. www.unicef.org/publications

Food for Thought: tackling child malnutrition to unlock potential and boost prosperity, Save the Children, 2013.

Handbook for emergencies. UNHCR/WHO. Geneva: WHO, 3rd edition. www.unhcr.org

Basic Virtual Library of Disaster Risk Management for Ministries of Health. WHO and PAHO (in CD format), 2013.

Mental health of refugees. UNHCR/WHO. Geneva: WHO, 1996.

Psychosocial Issues for Children and Families in Disasters. American Academy of Pediatrics Work Group on Disasters. US Department of Health and Human Services, 1995.

Red Book. American Academy of Pediatrics (AAP) Infectious Diseases Committee. AAP, 2012.

Refugee Children: determining the best interests of the child.
The United Nations High Commissioner for Refugees (UNHCR).
Geneva: UNHCR, 2008.

The Sphere Project: humanitarian charter and minimum standards
in disaster response – Sphere Training Package 2015.
www.sphereproject.org/news/new-sphere-training-materials

World Disaster Report. International Federation of Red Cross and
Red Crescent Societies, 2012.

THE WORLDWIDE WEB Helpful References

www.aap.org/new/disasterresources
American Academy of Pediatrics.

www.aap.org/terrorism/topics/psychosocial_aspects
American Academy of Pediatrics.

www.basics.org
E–mail: Infoctr@basics.org
Provides Basics Publications regarding child survival activities.

www.cdc.gov
The Centers for Disease Control Provides traveler's health
information, geographic health recommendations and disease
information.

www.cdmha.org
Center for Disaster Management and Humanitarian Assistance

www.dwb.org
Doctors without Borders (Médecins Sans Frontières (MSF)).

www.hvousa.org
Health Volunteers Overseas.

www.imva.org
The International Medical Volunteers Association provides
preparation resources for medical volunteers.

www.info.usaid.gov/hum_response

United States Agency for International Development.
Contains information from the Office for Foreign Disaster Assistance (OFDA), including the Field Operations Manual.

www.ipa-world.org
International Pediatrics Association.

www.oxfam.org

www.paho.org
Pan-American Health Organization provides information regarding the SUMA program, a system for planning and coordinating refugee needs.

www.reliefweb.int
Provides information on complex humanitarian emergencies, natural disasters and country backgrounds.

www.unhcr.ch
The United Nations High Commissioner for Refugees.

www.unicef.org
The United Nations Children's Fund.

Provides much relevant information, including the "Return to Happiness" program.

www.unv.org
United Nations Volunteers

www.who.int/eha/disasters/
WHO.

www.who.int/imci
WHO program on integrated management of childhood illness.

Made in the USA
San Bernardino, CA
02 December 2016